Extreme

Loss Hypnosis

The Proven Formula to Safe, Easy and Rapid Fat Loss. Regain Your Best Body Shape with Self-Hypnosis, Motivation, Guided Meditations and Gastric Band Hypnosis

Jennifer Young

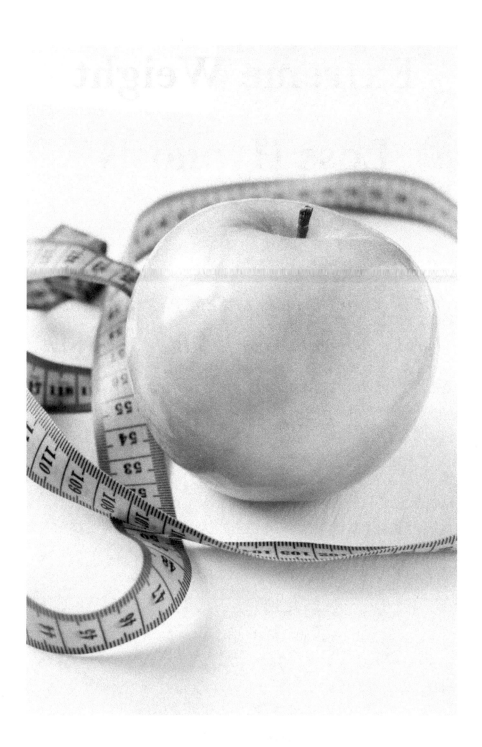

Table of Contents

Introduction

One of the most effective methods for achieving your objectives is hypnosis. It's a method that can be used for many different purposes, including weight loss. The goal in using hypnosis for weight loss is to create a new, positive frame of mind that will replace any previous thoughts that have been holding you back. Weight loss is a challenge for many people. They believe that losing weight and the stigma that comes with failure is difficult. Even more difficult is finding the motivation to work hard enough to shed those pounds. One of the things you can do with hypnosis is to change both your frame of mind and your motivation for losing weight. Here are three examples from three different sessions that will help you see how this works.

In this session, we combine hypnosis with guided meditation and gastric band hypnosis. The client has several medical problems, including high blood pressure and high cholesterol. She doesn't have a very good relationship with her own body. She feels that she is overweight. While in the session, she learns how to release these thoughts and feelings. In preparation for the session, we discuss the best type of hypnosis, what to wear and how to relax. We also discuss specific issues, such as her medical conditions, and address those issues during the session. The first goal is to help her focus on her health rather than on being fat or thin. That's why we start with an exercise that helps her release more negative feelings around food (gastric band hypnosis). We then move on to guided meditation, where she focuses on an aspect of her health that she truly enjoys (walking). We finish the session with a focus on gratitude and emotional freedom. She is thankful for the body she has and feels that way more often after the session.

In this session, we start with some baseline relaxation exercises to help her focus. Then we move into simple weight loss hypnosis, helping her visualize herself at a healthy weight, feeling good about her body and enjoying life with increased energy and less stress. We end by addressing fears related to food or food-related activities (gastric band hypnosis). This session specifically addresses her fears of not being able to maintain her weight at the new weight. We take these fears and turn them into an opportunity, rather than a reason for her to feel bad about herself. In this session, we combine weight loss hypnosis with guided imagination. The client is struggling with self-esteem issues around her body image. In the session, she learns that she can attain a wonderful level of self-confidence through hypnosis, and that she doesn't have to be fat or thin in order to feel good about herself. She learns how to use positive thinking and affirmation skills for weight loss as well. We also discuss feelings of anxiety and stress, and ways to address those feelings.

The new goal is to help her view herself as a valuable person, rather than as a less-than-perfect person. In this session, we combine weight loss hypnosis with guided fantasy. The client is struggling with high blood pressure and high cholesterol. She feels that her health problems are all related to her weight and doesn't know how to get better. In the session, she learns that there are three areas of her life in which she needs help with personal development: nutrition, fitness, and self-esteem (gastric band hypnosis). We teach her how to use hypnosis to do this and how she can use hypnosis to help herself feel good about herself. We also address some beliefs around weight loss and show her that she can be healthy at any weight. The goal is to help her accept that she can achieve weight loss success.

In all three of these sessions, we start with relaxation training so that the client will relax throughout the session. Then we move into a positive statements and mental exercises, as visualizations or affirmations. We conclude each session by reviewing the results from a relaxed state in which there were no negative feelings (e.g., gastric band hypnosis).

All three of these sessions, by themselves, would bring about change. However, the best way to use hypnosis is in combination with another methodology. For instance, you can combine weight loss hypnosis with gastric band hypnosis to help a client lose weight. You can combine it with guided meditation or guided imagery for positive thinking and self-esteem training. You can also combine it with guided fantasy for more advanced scenarios or for people who tend toward being more easily distracted.

What To Expect

Nothing is lost in these sessions. The client is always fully present and alert while in the session. You can expect a focused experience, where your client imagines herself at her goal weight, feeling good about her body and achieving success. If you want to go any further, we will discuss sophisticated simulation the methods or immersive imagery for particular scenarios.

How It Works

The tools that we use during hypnosis are relaxation training, positive statements, and mental exercises such as visualization or affirmations. In some cases, we may combine these methods with hypnosis. In others, we will move into more advanced techniques such as advanced visualization or more deliberate exercises for positive thinking (e.g. guided meditation). Most sessions are for weight loss and combine relaxation training with positive thoughts about weight loss. We start with a guided relaxation session in which the client learns to relax deeply using CBT techniques. Then we use simple positive statements along with mental exercises (visualization) related to weight loss.

When you combine the benefits of CBT and positive thinking, you get the best of both worlds. This combines the best of both worlds in a single session, helping your client relax and think about positive outcomes at the same time. As mentioned above, some sessions are for specific issues like anxiety or self-esteem. For these sessions, we will address specific issues and behaviors that go along with those issues (e.g. guided meditation, guided imagery, etc.). We will use visualization or affirmation sessions in each session to illustrate the tools that they need to overcome their issues.

Are You ready To Take the Next Step?

Now that you understand hypnosis and how we use it, it's time to learn about our weight loss hypnosis offerings. We have many different types of hypnosis for weight loss and we can accommodate most clients' requests. If you want a specific type of session (e.g. gastric band hypnosis), you can have it! If you just want an effective weight loss session, we can do that too! Our sessions are affordable and very easy to fit into your schedule. What are you waiting for? Don't you want to learn more about how our weight loss hypnosis sessions could help you lose weight faster and more effectively? Contact us today! We can't wait to hear from you!

Weight loss hypnosis is a proven method for helping people lose weight. It allows clients to reach higher levels of success faster than what they could do alone. By harnessing the power of the subconscious mind, people can focus on their goals and achieve them quickly. This not only helps people lose weight but allows them to keep the weight off permanently. Obesity prevention has long been advocated by dietary changes. While many people who are overweight or obese can lose some weight by changing what they eat, it's usually not enough to make a significant impact on their waistlines. In other words, dietary changes don't typically result in significant or permanent weight loss because they aren't supported by other lifestyle changes that are needed for long term results. You must concentrate on a lifestyle shift to lose weight and keep it off. Contact us today to learn more about how hypnosis will help you lose weight!

Dr. Clark has been a leading expert in using hypnosis for weight loss and health improvement for over 20 years. He currently teaches four training seminars per year to hundreds of people about how to use hypnotherapy effectively for weight loss, health improvement, and reduction of pain. Dr. Clark is a certified hypnotherapist who uses hypnosis to help clients achieve success. His primary goal is to teach people how to use hypnotherapy effectively and safely so they can experience extraordinary benefits of weight loss and improved health without any negative side effects.

Here are two real life examples of people who have used hypnosis successfully for weight loss: Eric was a 38-year-old father from Michigan whose inability to lose weight almost caused him to be diagnosed with diabetes before he finally took action by using the techniques, he learned through Dr. Clark's seminars. Here's what his story is like: "I've been following Dr. Clark's seminars for over a year. I started when I was almost at a point where I had to go on medication for my weight. My BMI was 42, which is overweight and almost the cutoff point for diabetes. Thanks to hypnosis, my BMI is now 38, which is within normal range."

Mandy was a 45-year-old woman from Texas who used hypnosis to lose 75 pounds and keep it off for six months! Here's her story: "I went through Dr. Clark's weight loss program in December of 2013. I lost 75 pounds total. I maintained the weight loss until June of 2014 and then started to gain back weight. Thanks to Dr. Clark's program, I'm now back on track and hoping to lose another 20 pounds by the end of the year." Both people simply changed their eating habits and used hypnosis for motivation. They didn't count calories or exercise to lose weight; they used a different method that works more efficiently than any other method available today. By using hypnosis, Eric and Mandy were able to change many areas of their lives at once in ways that are both sustainable and long lasting compared to more traditional methods.

Here's how hypnosis can help with weight loss. Hypnosis doesn't just allow you to lose weight and keep it off, it allows you to keep your healthy habits for the rest of your life as well! You'll have more success than you can imagine. Contact us today to get started with weight loss hypnosis! Weight loss is an intentional effort of a person to lose or shift from a defined amount of body mass. It is often used interchangeably with terms such as fat loss, or adiposity (the science of fat measurement and of the modeling). Other synonyms are lean mass gain, slimming, and hardening. In any case, weight loss can be achieved through energy intake and expenditure that is usually controlled by a diet. The term body mass gain refers to an increase in the body's mass. It can be used in a broad sense to mean loss of fat or muscle, or in a narrow sense to mean excessive growth of lean tissue. One example is exercise induced weight gain and muscle hypertrophy. Body builders often refer to this process as "bulking".

Also referred to as 'weight loss surgery' and 'recovery', there are many different reasons for wanting to lose weight. Although this procedure is very successful in helping to lose weight, there are risks involved which should be seriously considered before undergoing this type of surgery. It's worth noting that these dangers include not just the usual hazards of surgery, but also the possibility of medical complications linked to the surgical implants. As such, it is strongly advised that when choosing a weight loss procedure or preparation for surgery, you should seek recommendation and advice from a certified professional health care provider whose expertise correlates with your desires and goals.

Weight loss surgery often causes people to have 'carbohydrate rebound' (essentially an increase in muscle mass) after losing weight, possibly due to a change in hormonal balance overtime. This is of concern to many people who are trying to lose weight, as they are often advised that this is their body trying to regain weight lost through dieting, and as such should be avoided. Carbohydrate rebound occurs when there is an increase in muscle mass, due to a correlation between a rise in muscle mass and the amount of carbohydrates consumed.

Patients have access to a variety of weight loss services, some of which are listed on the National Health Service of the United Kingdom (NHS). In 2006, the NHS spent £43 million on obesity-related treatment, including bariatric surgery. The NHS Centre for Reviews and Dissemination (CRD) carried out a systematic review of 459 studies covering the effectiveness of various commercial, non-commercial, and complementary interventions. The conclusion was that 'Interventions aimed at losing weight or maintaining weight loss are more successful when components addressing psychological factors are included. Simple behavioural strategies to promote weight loss are unsuccessful and should therefore not be used as a component of most of these interventions. Weight loss is more effective when dietetic advice is provided by dietitians' (CRD, 2006).

Why People Fail to Lose Weight

What's the secret to weight loss? Certainly, there is no one-size-fits-all answer. But if you believe that your struggles with weight aren't simply related to overconsumption of calories -- but instead have more to do with internal factors, such as a skewed hormonal balance or emotional triggers like stress and anxiety -- then the hypnosis might be just the tool for you.

A recent poll revealed that 37% of respondents tried losing weight using some form of hypnosis (either self hypnosis or guided meditation) and found it helpful. Of those respondents, 50% said they lost a significant amount of weight. So How do Hypnosis and Weight Loss Connect? There are Two Primary Principles at Work Here:

1) Mind-Body Connection One of the most critical pieces of information you can get is the concept that your mind and body are connected. I know this may sound obvious, but what I mean by this is that not only does your mind influence your body -- it also influences other people's bodies! This means that there is a physical connection between you, other people, and their minds. At some level, everything is connected -- from the galaxies in outer space to the atoms in your body. Thus, it makes sense that when you think or do something, your physical cells know and respond to that. For example, let's say you are angry about an experience at work. Your body will react with increased heart rate, increased blood pressure and muscle tension. This stress response is the modern version of our "fight or flight" reaction from our caveman days when we were physically threatened by a saber-toothed tiger. Nowadays, most of us don't face imminent physical danger that often; however, many of us still have the same stress reaction to the day-to-day problems in life -- traffic jams and rude people at work, for example. The argument is that your thoughts and feelings have a physical response that you can control through simple self-hypnosis. If you imagine something to be greatly positive, your physical cells believe it -- or, at least, they aren't going to misbehave. The same concept applies if you are angry about an experience at work -- imagine the anger flowing away from your body along with the thoughts of what it and all its negative consequences could be doing to you.

2) Guided Visualization As we discussed above, when you think or do something, your mind knows and responds by making changes in your body. Therefore, I tell you to "visualize" things whenever possible -- it's not just to help your crayons draw better pictures, but it also helps your body. If you imagine yourself having a great time at a party, your physical cells begin making the transition to the party environment to prepare you for the event. The same idea applies with weight loss. People often struggle because they think about food all day and night -- not just when eating it. The result is that their bodies are convinced that they are starving and will step up their digestion and appetite behaviors into overdrive to deal with their "starvation." That's when using hypnotic techniques or guided visualization becomes critical. By imagining the food, you want to eat, in the right environment, your body will respond by accepting it as a gift and drawing it into your system.

Another example is if you imagine yourself having a wonderful relaxing meal, your physical cells will begin to relax and be in that same mindset. If this works for you, then imagine yourself walking outside at night and tricking your body by "dressing" in appropriate clothes for the occasion. The idea is not only to accept what you want to happen with regard to weight loss -- but also to be prepared for it by mentally preparing your body as well. This is the same concept that I teach in my weight-loss hypnotherapy sessions.

Eating Disorders Types

Are you recovering from an eating disorder? Are you looking for help to fight your inner demons? There are many different methods used to deal with eating disorders, but what are the best ones out there? Find out about several different eating disorder treatments and which ones will work best for you. Many have a long history of helping patients overcome their addictions, while others are entering the field for the first time.

Anorexia Nervosa- is an eating disorder marked by extreme weight loss, typically in women, and an abnormally low body weight. This behavior often involves severe dietary restrictions, excessive and/or compulsive exercise, and intensively focusing on body weight and shape to the exclusion of other interests. People with this disorder tend to see themselves as overweight even though they are extremely underweight. This behavior typically begins during teenage years or young adulthood.

Bulimia Nervosa- is an eating disorder characterized by binge eating accompanied by purging. Purging may include self-induced vomiting, misuse of laxatives or diuretics, and/or fasting. People with bulimia nervosa tend to cycle through periods of bingeing and purging. This behavior typically begins during teenage years or young adulthood.

Atkins Diet: The Atkins Diet has been controversial because of its restrictive nature. It is a very low-carbohydrate diet and emphasizes protein foods, such as meat and cheese. As you can imagine, this diet is not very balanced nutritionally because it lacks fresh vegetables, fruits, grains, etc.

Eating disorders are some of the most common mental illnesses in the world. They are characterized by repetitive behaviors that interfere with a person's nutritional and physical well-being. These behaviors may begin during adolescence or young adulthood, when one is under great pressure to look good or fit in. While eating disorders can affect anyone, they are more common in women and those who have experienced trauma in the past. Eating disorders such as bulimia nervosa and anorexia nervosa vary in etiology, nature, presentation, and treatment. The goal of treatment is to restore an individual's physical health while improving their understanding of their eating disorder so that they strive for a healthy lifestyle in the future. Eating disorders are complex conditions that require professional treatment to effectively manage symptoms and restore a patient's health. Treating anorexia nervosa is difficult because of the patient's desire to be thin. Anorexics typically deny that they have a problem and find treatment challenging. However, most can overcome the disorder with treatment and time. Most anorexics must continue with treatment on an outpatient basis to ensure their recovery is maintained or regained if they relapse. Anorexia nervosa can be successfully treated at most clinics using multidisciplinary approaches, which combine psychological therapy by trained experts in eating disorders with nutrition counseling.

Bulimia nervosa is usually treated on an outpatient basis, with the patient receiving treatment from a psychiatrist or psychologist. Many clinics also offer treatment programs for bulimia nervosa in order to provide patients with appropriate care. Treatment involves identifying the underlying causes of the disorder and learning healthy coping mechanisms to replace those that contribute to the development of unhealthy eating habits. However, bulimia nervosa may be treated in an inpatient facility if the patient has severe health complications due to their condition and is unable to maintain nutrition levels when attempting outpatient care.

Binge Eating Disorder: is characterized by binge eating large quantities of food in a short period of time on a regular basis (two hours). Binge eating is often accompanied by guilt and disgust or may lead to attempts at purging to decrease the feeling of being bloated after over-eating. People with binge eating disorder often experience mood swings, suicidal thoughts, and relationship problems that they believe are caused by their eating habits. Binge eating disorder can be successfully treated using a multidisciplinary approach, which combines counseling or therapy by a trained professional in the field of eating disorders.

Dopamine Medication: Dopamine is a neurotransmitter that helps brain cells communicate with one another; it plays an important role in the reward system of the brain. It is involved in many functions such as movement, sexual response, emotion and cognition. It is the neurochemical in the central nervous system that helps regulate movement and some of our other involuntary activities.

Dopamine has a long-lasting effect on an individual's behavior and moods; without it, people may experience giddiness, loss of motor control, emotional numbness, a lack of motivation and reduced concentration. Patients with Parkinson's disease have decreased dopamine activity in the brain which can result in problems controlling movements. Treatment for these patients can also include certain medications that increase dopamine activity.

Treating a patient with ADHD may require increasing their levels of dopamine so that they are more able to complete tasks or concentrate on difficult tasks. The use of ADHD medication may be necessary to help improve functioning in patients with a dopamine deficiency. Certain dopamine-increasing medications can also be used.

Eating disorders are some of the most common mental illnesses in the world. They are characterized by repetitive behaviors that interfere with a person's nutritional and physical well-being. These behaviors may begin during adolescence or young adulthood, when one is under great pressure to look good or fit in. Eating disorders such as bulimia nervosa and anorexia nervosa vary in etiology, nature, presentation and treatment.

The American Psychiatric Association has identified five distinct eating disorders, including anorexia nervosa, bulimia nervosa, the binge eating disorder (BED), the problem-eating category and the pica disorder. Although anorexia is generally considered a life-threatening disorder, it is often most difficult to treat. Treatment for the other four disorders may be more effective and less draining on both professional and personal levels.

Nowadays, obesity and other related weight problems have become such a common health issue that it is considered a worldwide epidemic. This book is for you if you're one of the millions of people who suffer from this issue. It's for people who want to lose weight quickly without the pain and suffering that other dieters experience. We introduce some of the most popular extreme weight loss methods being used today – hypnosis, guided meditation, and gastric band hypnosis.

Why do people suffer from eating disorders in the first place? There are many reasons for this, but one of the most common is that they are constantly exposed to media messages and images which promote the glorification of being overweight. For example, if you take a look at almost any Hollywood actress, you will find that they are practically overweight – in fact it's considered fashionable.

These messages have an extremely damaging effect on the self-esteem and self-worth of a lot of people. Studies have been done which show that modeling and media images of overly thin women can actually cause some young women to develop eating disorders like anorexia nervosa in order to try and attain the ideal of beauty that they see promoted all around them every day. It's so easy for teenagers or young adults to slip into these negative thought patterns, especially if their self-confidence is lower than normal.

In order to combat this issue, a hypnotherapist can help you get to the root of your problem. She or he can then use hypnosis, guided meditation, or gastric band hypnosis to rewire your brain and reprogram it with positive affirmations that will make you become more confident about your body image. This will help you avoid all other issues related to obesity such as depression, anxiety, etc. Let's now take a look at some of the most effective treatments available today.

Extreme Weight Loss Hypnosis: Extreme weight loss hypnosis is one of the most popular methods used for dealing with obesity. This type of therapy will help you gain trust and self-esteem while also increasing your knowledge of your own body image. Through hypnosis, you'll be able to get rid of all the mental and emotional barriers that have been holding you back from reaching your ideal weight. It doesn't matter if you're already obese or just slightly overweight, these sessions can still help you achieve your goals without having to go through pain or suffering. It's amazing how such a simple therapy can change your life completely.

GUIDE MEDITATION & GASTRIC BAND HYPNOSIS: This is another kind of treatment that is specifically designed for dealing with obesity and related issues. In this type of therapy, a specialist will guide you through guided meditation and gastric band hypnosis sessions that are specifically designed for people who have recently chosen to lose weight. The hypnotherapist is not a miracle worker and you won't find yourself losing a lot of weight immediately after the first session. However, you'll notice that your cravings for sweets and other fatty foods will start to disappear gradually. In addition, these treatments will make you more aware of your natural hunger cues and how to satisfy them with healthier meals, rather than eating until you're completely stuffed. In addition, you'll also be able to appreciate your body more, rather than being too obsessed with it and trying to change it. Trust yourself and be persistent and you'll soon start seeing all the positive changes that you've always wanted. Losing weight is often a difficult task. But it's not impossible. These three hypnosis downloads may be the answer you've been looking for whether you're looking to lose weight or just maintain a healthy weight.

1) Extreme Weight Loss Hypnosis - This is one of the most effective ways to help yourself achieve your weight-loss goals in a safe and healthy manner. When you have this type of session with an experienced professional, there's no need to suffer through harsh "diets" or "crash" programs that are difficult to stick with long term. You can learn to eat in moderation and establish a healthy lifestyle that fits your needs.

2) Guided Meditation - This meditation download is great for anyone but is especially helpful for those individuals who are struggling with an addiction. If you're looking to become free from alcohol or other drugs,

hypnosis might be the right solution. Just make sure that you choose a program that is geared toward helping you overcome a specific addiction, such as smoking cessation hypnosis or alcoholism hypnosis.

3) Gastric Band Hypnosis - This type of program helps individuals create a mental "band" (much like an actual gastric band) around their waistline. The program helps them associate a "healthy" weight with a particular body part. This band helps people change their behaviors and thoughts, which leads to a quicker and more effective weight loss effort. But remember you have to dedicate yourself to the program. These programs are not going to "do it all for you." It takes consistent work, consistency, and commitment from both you and your doctor. But if managed properly, this type of program can help you achieve your goals in a safe, healthy way.

The Right Mindset to Have on Weight Loss Diet

No Matter what type of weight loss diet you have, the most important thing is your mindset. You need to make sure that you have the right attitude and mental outlook on eating less and exercising more. Otherwise, you will end up quitting before it gets off the ground. In order to stick with your weight loss diet, it's important for you to start by 'feeling' good about yourself when you start losing weight. Don't get caught up in temporary problems, such as how you feel about your body. Focus instead on how good you feel about losing weight because of the energy it gives you.

The next thing to consider is that your willpower is the most important part of your weight loss diet success. You have to give up many things during weight loss, including food and other activities that you enjoy. You can't just skip them or eat them in secret when no one is watching you. Instead, make sure that you are giving it all up for a purpose and believing that it will lead to something bigger than yourself. That's what "willpower" is all about, you have to really believe in yourself and your diet plan. Try to keep a positive attitude. Don't tell yourself that you can't have something or that food is bad for you. Instead, look at it as a 'special thing' that will help get you in the right frame of mind to achieve your goal weight. You want to make sure that you keep everything positive and happy so that your weight loss diet and exercise program works the way it's supposed to work!

Limit time for eating and drinking as much as possible. This will keep you from eating mindlessly, and it will force you to realize when you're full. For example, if you have a half hour to pick the kids up from school or take them to their activities, you should limit yourself to a can of soda and one cookie. This will prevent you from eating more while driving.

Keep in mind that it's often easier for some people lose weight than others. Just because someone seems like they have everything straight doesn't mean that they are doing well with a weight loss diet. Take the feedback of your friends and family seriously, but don't jump into believing the lies that other people try to spread about your "illness" or "diet problem". You're working hard to lose weight, so be proud of yourself for doing well!

Weight Loss Hypnosis: The Secrets to Lose Weight Quickly

Does hypnosis work for weight loss? It might. But you don't have to spend a lot of money on expensive spa treatments, or even on more books and videos about how you can make the change and lose weight. Instead, you can get the tools you need right here and right now with hypnosis downloads. Everything is available at a very low price. When looking for tools that can help you make changes in your life, remember that it is important to find out what is behind those feelings. If you want the hypnosis to help you lose weight, you should talk with a trained specialist who can help you get at the heart of why you want to change, and then make those changes in your life. Of course, the special programs that are offered online today mean that it is now easy to find information that can help you get quality tools to help you get the results that you want.

First thing's first: Before using anything for weight loss, talk with your doctor about any issues or concerns that might be related to hypnotherapy or other treatments. Then listen to some sample recordings online and see if they are right for your situation. You need to find out whether they work for your goals and needs.

Next, make sure that you understand how the program works. There are many types of downloads that can be used for weight loss, and each of them might have a different purpose and process. Some are more helpful for losing weight quickly, while others might be better for making lasting changes in your life so that you can sustain your progress for years to come. You need to understand the process to know how it will work for you. Finally, make sure that you put the program into effect as soon as possible so that you can see results fast. This will help you keep up your motivation to continue on with your new program. You want to get something that works for you and that will help you live a healthier life, so don't hesitate to find out more about how this type of program can make a difference in your life.

You can lose weight in a number of ways. Diet and exercise are one way to do it, and hypnosis downloads are another. Many people wonder whether or not hypnosis for weight loss is the right option for them, but it really depends on the individual and the results they want to see with their body. Weight loss hypnosis does work for some people, but not necessarily all of them.

Many people do not understand how hypnosis works for weight loss, but it really is a great way to help you get the results that you want. If you are looking for a way to change your body, hypnosis can be the way for this to happen. It can help you make lasting changes in your life so that you will see results that last for years to come. Whether or not weight loss hypnosis is right for everyone, it does work well for many people who want to lose weight and see lasting results in all areas of their lives.

One of the best things about weight loss hypnosis is that it is very affordable and easy to use. Many people use it on a regular basis, and they can make lasting changes in their lives that will help them live a healthier life. Find out more about the process of hypnosis for weight loss to find out how it can really help you.

Weight Loss Hypnosis: Why It Works So Well

The most beneficial aspect of hypnosis is that it will assist you while you are operating alone. You do not need someone else to help you with the process; instead, hypnosis allows you to focus on yourself and your goals, helping you make lasting changes in your life so that you can have a better future because of it.

Weight loss hypnosis also works well because it offers options that can last for years. This program does not have to be limited to a set number of months or days. Instead, it can help you achieve the best benefits for the long term.

It's important for you to understand all of your options when it comes to weight loss hypnosis. There are many different types of hypnosis recordings available today that help people make changes in their lives. Some may offer additional features as well, so it is important for you to learn which one works best for you and your needs.

As you continue to learn more about weight loss hypnosis, you will find that you are better able to make an educated decision. Make sure that you take the time to find out everything that you need to know about this option so that it can help with your weight loss goals.

There are lots of different options for anyone who wants to lose weight. This form of hypnosis has been known to work well in the past, and with the recent advances in technology, it is even better now than it once was. Make sure that you find a program that appeals to your needs and fits into your life as well as possible. This will give you a chance at success without much effort on your part. The best way to get a thorough understanding of weight loss hypnosis is to learn all you can. Make sure that you take the time to understand what it can do for you, as well as any potential risks that might be involved in trying this method. After you know all of this, you will be better off deciding whether or not this is the right option for your needs. For anyone who is looking for results with weight loss hypnosis, there are lots of different things that they should take into account. Make sure that you learn about everything involved with this method, and then make an informed decision on whether or not this is something that could help with your goals.

My way of tracking my goals is by taking pictures of various scenes and objects in nature. I call them "goals" because it helps me to see what I really want to do. For example, the photo above shows a sand dune on the beach with lots of shells and broken seashells on the ground. Now, I don't care about shells; over time this scene has become commonplace to me and I don't think about it as much anymore. It doesn't matter if it is good or bad for my goals, but it has become something that doesn't move me emotionally in any way that changes my level of motivation towards getting closer to achieving them.

My goal is to do things that can be called "good", but I don't necessarily think that they are good for me or the world. This way of thinking is a good way to look at my goals. What is important is how it makes me feel, and not what it does for everyone else in the world. I am not sure if this philosophy will work for everyone who wants to take better care of themselves and get in shape. My way of doing things may be very different from some people's methods of making healthier changes in their lives. When people ask me what I do to lose weight and eat healthier, I tell them that I take pictures of my goals... it seems to confuse them. In fact, some of the things that are important to me are not healthy at all. For all they know about my goals, they may think that I am a crazy person who is obsessed with sand dunes and broken seashells. It is not true, but it doesn't matter when it comes to these things.

Sand dunes are a type of scenery or landscape for me, and so are shells on the ground. I love taking pictures of things like this because it reminds me of my goals and what I want to accomplish. It is so wonderful that I can get the emotions out of my system and express them in such a way.

I do not need to eat healthier or lose weight for any reason other than that I would like to look better in the clothes that I wear and feel better about myself. This philosophy works really well for me, but it may not work for everyone else.

If you have goals for yourself, you should consider putting the pictures of them somewhere where you will be able to see them often. Maybe you can get a nice frame for your goal post and put it up on your wall. You should take photographs of the scenery around you and use them as reminders of your objectives.

I think that people should be able to make healthier changes in their lives, even if they don't like or want to do it. People should be able to make changes in their lives that help improve their health on a whole, though this might not always happen.

I find it better to think of your goals as something that you can do for yourself. People should only do things that are good for them, even if it means that they have to give up other things on a whole. I think that people should only want the best for themselves, even if it means that other people might not want what is best for themselves. You should only go through with something that will help you feel better about yourself on a whole. You do not have to go through life being miserable and uncomfortable because it is what other people want or because they are trying to be healthy and fit into their clothing. You can only realize your goals if you are healthy enough to pursue them without being miserable about the process.

It is important for people to know that they can make changes in their lives if they really want them badly enough. Some people might not care about themselves, but they should want the best for themselves anyway. You won't have to think about anything because you'll only be able to make changes in your life that help others around you as well as yourself.

Importance Of Self-Love, Self-Esteem And Self-Acceptance

Importance of self-love, self-esteem and self-acceptance:

People who don't like their body and are unhappy with the way they look tend to make less healthy decisions in their day-to-day lives. One study by the National Institutes of Health found that people who are dissatisfied with their bodies and feel shame about themselves are more likely to smoke, drink alcohol, eat unhealthy foods and not exercise. There is a very common notion that one needs willpower in order to stay inspired and motivated enough for life changes. But as you can see this is not true at all! Willpower is something we all have, but it's simply not always easy to access when you're feeling stressed, downhearted or discouraged. I know how hard it is to stay positive and motivated when you are in that state of mind, so I have made it my goal to help you change your mindset.

I believe that with hypnosis we can change our mindset into a more optimistic one without the use of willpower, simply by tapping into the power of the subconscious mind. The subconscious mind is where our core beliefs are stored and where we can access unlimited power when in a relaxed state. It is also for that reason that it's very easy to change old thought patterns and adopt new ones in an instant while under hypnosis. As a certified Hypnosis instructor I have learned how to tap into this unlimited source of power. It's a simple procedure done in two parts. The first part is the induction, which is exactly what it sounds like. It's an easy 5 minute process where you can go deeper and deeper as you go under until you reach the level of trance. And once you are there your subconscious mind will start telling you all kinds of fantastic stories that will enable you to make the changes that you want to make in your life!

The second part of the process is what I call "visualization" technique. This step involves the use of guided imagery. In the visualization step you will visualize how your future self looks while listening to my voice guiding you. This is an amazing part of the process because, again, by changing your mindset you will unconsciously change your future self for the better.

As a Certified Hypnotist, I have helped hundreds of people lose weight and keep it off through hypnosis and hypnosis-related products.

It's no mystery that the more you care for yourself, the better your health. And if you've ever set foot in a gym, seen an advertisement on TV, or checked out a diet book at the library, then you're already aware of this. But what if there was another way? One that focuses exclusively on what's best for you: your heart, your mind and your soul?

This is where health hypnosis comes in. Health hypnosis is a gentle, drug-free process that utilizes the power of your subconscious mind to help you make positive changes that last. With the assistance of hypnosis, you can change your lifestyle, overcome obstacles and improve your appearance—without having to alter the way you live. And best of all? With health hypnosis, there's no limit to how far you can reach! Weight loss hypnosis may be just that way! Hypnosis allows people to reach deeply into their subconscious mind where they can learn to lose weight in a way that will be long lasting. The gastric band hypnosis is also helpful as it helps one feel full sooner and controls appetite. The weight loss hypnosis will help one to learn how to love themselves again.

Importance of Self-Love:

Self-love is the key to progress. When you love yourself, you don't want to sabotage yourself with bad eating habits and poor health choices. Your mind and body are connected in more ways than one – and while your thoughts may have a direct impact on your health, you also have control over your thinking process. You can train your mind to think healthier if you practice positive affirmations on a daily basis. This allows your subconscious mind to accept them as true. Self-love is obviously a very difficult thing to achieve. But it is completely possible. It will take time and it takes work, but the results are always worth it.

How to Start Loving Yourself:

As someone who has unfulfilled weight loss goals in the past, I am committed to achieving them and learning what it truly means to care for myself. It can be difficult at times but I learned to stop looking for external things like diet pills and weight loss programs to make me feel like I am good enough – because of course, I am not!

Hypnosis is a safe technique through which one can start loving and accepting themselves – no matter how difficult it is. Guided meditation is even better and allows the mind to carry out the instructions given during it. This is when one may be able to truly experience the deep love for oneself and the passion for everything else that comes along with it. The inner energy can also be focused on a particular goal. This helps in getting rid of all negative thoughts, which are usually what hold us back. Hypnosis is a great tool that can be used by weight loss experts to help their patients as well as individuals who want to get rid of negative thoughts permanently.

How To Improve Your Self-Love:

The first step would be to put in the effort that is necessary to reach this goal in the first place. You don't need an intense workout session every day or hours of cardio or kickboxing (unless you're already doing it). You just need to start doing things that are good for your body, such as exercise, yoga and massage. There are also several books about mindfulness and positive thinking which can help you learn how to love yourself and improve it over time.

If you're finding it difficult to start loving yourself and taking better care of yourself, you can try doing some self hypnosis and positive affirmations. Doing this will allow you to become more aware of all the things that you love about your body, including the weight loss it has caused. You can use the "Affirmations for Weight Loss" book to help you address these things.

You need to remind yourself of all the things that are good about your body, for example your hair and skin as well as muscles and everything else that makes up your perfect body. You can also use affirmations to focus on all the good things that you have done in life so far. This can help you stay motivated as well as continue loving yourself, no matter what.

It is very important that you still remind yourself of all the things that aren't good about yourself because this will help with self acceptance. You need to realize that it's not about the weight loss itself, but about changing your thoughts and feelings on the topic and loving yourself for who you are now. At first, it may be best to start with techniques like visualizations and affirmations as they will be quite helpful.

However, when you notice that your positive emotions are increasing and that you are becoming more accepting of yourself, then it's time to switch to self love hypnotherapy. This will help you to get even stronger feelings of self love and acceptance in the long term. It involves setting up a schedule for your sessions and following it every day or every week.

This also means that you will have plenty of opportunities to start practicing positive affirmations any time during the day. This way, you can use them whenever you want, especially if some negative thoughts appear about yourself or your weight loss. However, the more that you practice them in the context of hypnosis, the better results will come along with it as well.

Therefore, start practicing them in the morning and at night, when you are activated with your emotions. You will also find that sometimes you are already starting to feel more positive emotions towards yourself without even trying. This is because your subconscious mind can sense a change in your mental state. It adjusts its thoughts towards you as well.

This is why practices like self-hypnosis can be so effective in changing your actions and moods towards you positively as well as for long term effects. The best thing about it is that it doesn't matter if hypnotherapy is something that you want to do regularly or only once or twice a week. If you are properly trained, then you can move at your own pace. This makes it a very successful way of dealing with any problems that may be bothering you in your life.

Of course, many people will want to see how it works out for them in order to see whether they would like to continue going down this path. The problem is that it is very expensive and many people find that they cannot afford to get a session regularly. However, that doesn't mean that you should just take the first offer of a free hypnotherapy session that you get from an unqualified therapist. The problem is that the therapist may not really care about what you want and what your level of experience is in this new field. You need to find someone who isn't just good at hypnotherapy but also someone who is experienced and qualified in dealing with weight loss.

You can find this type of therapy in most clinics or health centers. However, you should also check online to see if you can find something that is more suitable for your needs. This way, you will have a chance to find something that is cheaper than the offline sessions and you may be able to get a good deal on it in order to help save money. Also, this way allows you to get a session whenever you like, without having to wait for someone who is qualified enough to give it in your area.

If you want to use self-hypnosis to help you change your lifestyle and achieve a better balance, then I recommend that you first of all learn more about it. You can also decide whether or not you want to pursue it on your own so that you do not depend on anyone else for your happiness. This way, it's just up to you and nobody else!

In the end, if you want to know the best way to make self love and acceptance a part of your life permanently, then you should definitely look into hypnotherapy sessions and using them on a daily basis. This is something that can be very beneficial for your ongoing weight loss journey so try it out today.

Rewriting Brain: How to Overcome Weight Loss Limiting Beliefs

Do you feel like you have tried everything? Do you worry that other people can tell what size clothes to buy by looking at your shape? Are you tired of feeling confined in the world due to your weight when it is something over which you have absolutely no control? We'll look at three different forms of brain rewriting in this book: hypnosis, guided meditation, and gastric band hypnosis. These are all safe and effective ways to change your beliefs about food and weight loss while interacting with a therapist trained in these techniques.

Overcoming Weight Loss Limiting Beliefs with Hypnosis

Changing our eating values is the first step toward changing our eating habits. The only way we can truly have the weight loss we want and deserve is if we believe it's possible and adjust our expectations about what will happen when. However, if you've tried hypnosis before or are even a little nervous about the whole thing, you might be wondering how safe it really is. First of all hypnosis is much safer than you might think. In fact, whether or not hypnosis will work for you depends on your expectations of what hypnotherapy actually entails. When we're in a hypnotic state, our ability to be aware of reality is reduced – including our awareness of pain. For this reason many people think they can't be hypnotized when they really can. But even if you fear hypnosis, it's still possible to work with your therapist in a safe and effective manner.

How Does Hypnosis Work?

Hypnosis works through suggestion. When you're in hypnosis, your mind begins to play along with the ideas that are being presented to you through the deep stimulation and directed visualization processes. You might think of it as something like dreaming, except you're awake and fully aware. The goal is to change your beliefs, behaviors, and habits that are standing in your way of a healthier you through suggestion rather than willpower.

When you are hypnotized for weight loss purposes, your hypnotherapist will work with you on changing your belief systems about food and weight loss. The goal is to transform negative or unhealthy beliefs into positive ones that support healthy eating choices and healthy body image.

Is Hypnosis the Only Method?

Most people are familiar with guided visualization and guided meditation as methods associated with hypnosis. Many therapists also use the imagery skills learned in an art therapy class as part of their work with clients. Even those who do not utilize hypnosis often use many of the same techniques through guided imagery. Some therapists like to include more traditional ways of helping clients work through their weight loss issues, such as behavior modification therapies or other counseling approaches. Your therapist will be able to tell you what approach they prefer based on your goals and what they feel will best benefit you. If you've tried hypnosis before and it didn't function for you, it's possible that your expectations were the issue. If you're nervous about trying it again, remember that most successful sessions involve between 5-15 minutes of true hypnosis. Even if your therapist does choose hypnosis as a method to work with you, they might also incorporate other techniques to complement their work. Using multiple methods can give you the best results possible and help you permanently overcome unhealthy beliefs about food and weight loss before they become a problem in your everyday life.

Changing Your Brain to Change your Body

So how can changing your thoughts and beliefs about food and weight loss help you achieve the body you want? It's simple. When you have healthy, positive beliefs about the food you eat, it becomes much easier to make healthy choices. For example, if you believe that eating a piece of pizza will make you fat and miserable, then that's probably exactly what will happen. However, if you know that eating a pizza every once in a while won't change the way your body looks or feels (and doesn't make every day pizza night), then there's no reason not to indulge yourself sometimes.

During a typical session of hypnosis the therapist will have you enter a state of deep relaxation while giving suggestions to increase your awareness of these beliefs. Here are some examples of the types of changes you might experience:

Believing that your body is not too large.

Noticing that you have a high metabolism that allows you to eat more food and still lose weight. Letting go of the idea that exercise must be hard or painful in order to have an effect on your weight. Understanding that healthy eating does not require deprivation. It can be pleasurable and relaxing. The goal of hypnosis for weight loss is to help you notice beliefs and patterns of thinking that stand in the way of healthy eating habits while constructing new, healthier ones. There is no need for willpower or self-control here because these changes are made through suggestion rather than external force. "I understand that one of the major reasons for low self-esteem is due to negative thoughts about being overweight. I can choose not to believe these negative thoughts, knowing that they are created from fear and insecurity. Instead, I can choose to believe in my beauty and value as a human being."

Do You Need Hypnosis For Weight Loss or Weight Loss Surgery?

If you are looking for hypnosis for weight loss surgery, there is no need to panic. This type of hypnotherapy is not for everyone. If you are seeking this type of therapy because you have come across conflicting information online about whether or not it works, I assure you it does work for most people. If you're the type of person who is eager to get started on your weight loss surgery journey, then hypnosis should be the next step, not a substitute for weight loss surgery. If you are seeking hypnosis for weight loss but haven't yet had gastric bypass or another weight loss procedure, then it would likely be a good idea to have hypnotherapy before surgery. However, if you are already in recovery from your gastric banding procedure or gastric bypass, I'd recommend waiting at least 6 months before seeking out therapeutic hypnotherapy. This is not to say that hypnosis can't be effective after your surgery. In fact, many people do benefit from this type of therapy and it can help you make the most of your weight loss surgical procedure.

How Can Hypnotherapy Help Me?

The best part about working with a trained hypnotherapist on your weight loss journey is that they will guide you through a process that lets you find the answers on your own. They will suggest certain things and then allow you the opportunity to come up with your own conclusions based on these suggestions. Your weight loss journey will be tailored specifically to you and your needs.

You can also expect hypnosis to enhance other weight loss techniques that you are already using. For example, if you are already working with a nutritionist and following a healthy eating plan, hypnotherapy could be used in conjunction with this in order to reinforce your new learning and help keep you on track. Hypnotherapy will also improve your overall quality of life, not just your physical health. You'll have more positive self-esteem and be more confident in yourself – making it easier to maintain the changes you make over time.

Our Hypnotherapist's Weight Loss Journey

In 2008, I began my weight-loss journey. I was in my early thirties and fifty pounds overweight. At the time, I had a stressful job, low self-esteem and no energy. Like most people who are overweight, I believed that I would be "skinny" if I lost enough weight or ate the right foods or exercised enough. I tried numerous diets, pills and programs without success. So even though hypnosis didn't work for me at first (it seemed like it did, but it stopped working after awhile), that didn't deter me from trying it again a few years later. I knew that I had to find something that worked, so I was willing to try anything at this point.

I had a consultation with a licensed psychotherapist about five years after my first meeting. She was also my counselor during my weight loss surgery. After practicing hypnotherapy with her, I started seeing a hypnotherapist on my own in early 2015 – the same year I had gastric bypass surgery. She has been assisting me in regaining my health for the past year and a half, which has been a constant struggle for me. But now it's the first time in 4 years that I have felt normal again. My energy is back and I haven't been sick in over a year. I'm not perfect, but I feel great and am continuing to work towards my goals.

My weight loss journey isn't over – it will never be over – but now that I have the tools and skills to help myself, it has become much easier. Hypnotherapy has changed my life and continues to change my life for the better! Hypnosis will assist you in investing in your own success if you are able to do so. You won't find a more upbeat, encouraging environment than 12Keys Hypnosis Center.

I did some research and learned that hypnotherapy wasn't just for people with weight issues. It could also be used for anxiety and depression, and to improve memory – so I decided to try it again in 2011. This time, I dropped over 100 pounds in less than a year with the help of a hypnotist. I was able to quit smoking by quitting cold turkey using self-hypnosis. I was also able to use hypnosis when dealing with periods of anxiety or depression and found that it helped me overcome my negative thoughts surrounding these things.

Part of my weight loss journey included a change in diet/nutrition to include these things that I picked up using hypnosis. For example, I learned how to make better food choices based on what I really wanted rather than my perceived or perceived outdated ideas about what was right for me. This may sound very strange, but it's true – and it works! (Much like the way hypnosis works!)

I found that being able to tap into my subconscious mind helped me achieve all kinds of amazing things! Knowing that every time I ate something, it affected me physically also helped motivate me to make better food choices. And although I didn't use self-hypnosis to quit smoking, it was a huge help in my battle to quit. I downloaded a hypnosis program that helped me quit by helping me relax and slow my breathing. Another "side effect" of this effort was that I began sleeping better and waking up without an alarm! Another "side effect" of quitting smoking was that I also lost weight! I started noticing that my clothes were getting looser as I lost the excess weight.

I'm certain that had I continued smoking, I would have continued to gain weight and struggle to lose it - but with hypnosis, I was able to begin to transform my own behaviors (including those surrounding food), and this is what helped me reach my goal. And although the weight never did come off like it did initially, at least now I was no longer trying to "will" it off because I knew it would never happen if I did not focus on making healthy choices around food.

Today, I am in my 40s and much healthier than when I was in my 20s. It's never fun to be overweight – but it doesn't have to be a permanent condition. With the right tools and mindset, you can change it too!

What Happens During a Hypnosis For Weight Loss Session?

During a hypnosis for weight loss session, your therapist will talk with you about your goals and development points. They will ask questions about how you feel and what aspects of yourself you feel would benefit from changing within yourself. In addition, they will determine what needs to be changed within you in order for you to achieve your goal weight; or if you have already achieved it, they will make recommendations on how to maintain it. A set of questions can be asked by your therapist during this period. These questions are designed to help find out more about your self-image and what is holding you back from attaining the body that you want and deserve. Questions may include:

What ideas, beliefs, and attitudes are you having about your own body? Are those ideas consistent with the way that you've treated yourself in the past?

Are there positive thoughts or rules that you have about your own body? If so, where did those come from? What are they like?

Hypnosis is a form of psychological counseling that is different than therapy in that it is more focused on helping clients reach bottom-line results. Often referred to as self-hypnosis or auto-suggestion, a hypnotist uses inductive techniques and other tools to assist clients with overcoming habits and behaviors that hinder their potential for achieving goals. Hypnosis is effective for many different modalities, including weight loss. If you are looking to shed unwanted pounds and maintain a healthy lifestyle, hypnosis can be an effective tool for changing your behaviors around food. It will help you incorporate healthy habits into your normal routines, so that you will be able to maintain them. How can hypnotherapy support weight loss? Hypnosis can help support weight loss by helping clients with goal setting and by eliminating the feelings of guilt and self-blame that often accompany diets and exercises programs. Hypnosis encourages the ideas of self-acceptance and self-love, which in many ways are necessary prerequisites for permanent weight loss. Hypnosis also can empower an individual by helping them identify their true potential, motivating them to greater success.

How To Overcome Emotional Eating

Oh, emotional eating. We've all been there: the stress-induced binge, the momentary ease you find in a chocolate bar, or an entire cake consumed in one sitting. We enjoy it while we're doing it and regret it later when our stomachs feel sore and bloated.

It may sound counterproductive, but hypnotherapy can be an effective way to manage your emotional eating. In fact, some hypnosis sessions for weight loss include the use of hypnotic techniques to help your mind heal itself from emotional eating and other addictions. Oral hypnotherapy, which involves having a hypnotist speak directly in your ear, may be most comfortable for you - but this method is often costly and not always covered by insurance. This simple how-to guide will teach you the basics of how to get started with hypnotherapy for weight loss. Start reading now so that you can overcome emotional eating later today!

The Preeminent Step Is To Have A Goal

Recognize that there is nothing inherently wrong with emotional eating. Emotional eating is nothing more than taking out your emotional baggage to relieve stress. However, if you want to stop it from becoming a habit, there must be a way to do so.

Step 1: In overcoming emotional eating is to have a goal. Whether it's dropping ten pounds in one week or getting into better shape, the act of having a goal allows you to focus on the task at hand instead of just giving into unhealthy cravings

Step 2: Dissect Your Eating Habits To Identify The Emotional Eating Link

No matter what your goal, looking at the steps of how you eat can help identify when you are emotionally eating. Consider these questions: When do you eat? Do you ever feel sad, lonely, or stressed in a specific time of the day? Do you eat a certain food to help yourself feel better? What triggers your cravings? Being aware of your eating habits will help remind you to avoid emotional eating.

Step 3: Use Hypnosis For Weight Loss To Let Go Of Emotional Eating

As I mentioned earlier, hypnotherapy can be one way of dealing with emotional eating. However, this may not be an affordable option. In fact, some forms of hypnosis for weight loss are so expensive that they cost more than weight loss surgery! If this is your case, then there are other techniques that you can use at home.

Do you turn to junk food when you're feeling down or stressed out? Do your emotions get the better of you? Would you like to change that for good? Hypnosis is a powerful tool for personal transformation. These amazing hypnosis audio recordings are designed to help anyone stop and lose weight without dieting, pills, or deprivation. You'll be able to make the permanent changes in your eating habits and emotional well-being that have escaped your efforts before. Within a few minutes, you can achieve immediate results in your eating and lifestyle habits. More than just another weight loss product, our hypnosis downloads are the only tools you'll need to achieve your goals. Simply download them and listen as often as you like.

Step 4: Apply Cognitive Behavioral Therapy To Overcome Emotional Eating
Cognitive behavioral therapy (CBT) is an effective way to address emotional eating issues. This method focuses on helping people learn to identify and correct their thought patterns that lead to unhealthy behaviors, such as overeating emotionally. Although anyone can benefit from CBT, those with eating disorders may want to consider working with a clinical psychologist who can assist them in developing a non-confrontational approach that is in line with their treatment philosophy.

Step 5: Look At Your Lifestyle To See What Triggers Your Emotional Eating
So you're trying to stop an emotional eating habit, but every time your friend calls you, you feel powerless and helpless. Or maybe you eat when you're upset about something at work or home. Regardless, understanding where the trigger is coming from is the key to overcoming it. In many cases, a change of diet may be in order after identifying the cause behind your emotional eating. For example, if you are prone to overeating when stressed and have a co-worker that constantly criticizes your work, then reducing workplace stress may be beneficial for overcoming the behavior pattern.

Step 6: Watch Your Emotions Rather Than Food

Your emotions are not the enemy; they are simply part of your life. When you give yourself a moment to take a break and sit down and think about how you're feeling, it's possible to focus on what you're upset about rather than on the food in your stomach. We often think food is an escape when we're feeling stressed or sad, but it's easy for us to get caught in the cycle of emotional eating. However, when you take a moment to dwell on your emotions, then take action by giving yourself an alternative coping strategy to solve problems, there is a chance that you may find your way out of this trap.

Step 7: Find Your Emotional Eating Price Tag
When you're emotionally eating, it's easy to let the negative emotions overtake your ability to make rational decisions. However, knowing how much you've spent on your unhealthy behaviors can help you begin to put a price tag on each emotional eating episode.

If there are other ways that you can solve the problem without consciously plugging into the food, then focus on those instead. For example, if a co-worker is always complaining about you and you feel like there's no recourse for them to get better management skills, then helping them learn will benefit everyone involved in the situation.

So, What's the Solution?

Whether you're looking to lose weight, stop smoking, or get a better handle on your emotions and more, nutrition and psychotherapy are two of the most commonly recommended solutions. However, hypnosis can provide you with the tools necessary to look at your habits in a new light.

When you understand how those habits work in your brain and how they originate, then you can begin to change the way that you eat through education and understanding. You'll no longer feel like you have to turn to unhealthy foods when you're stressed or upset; instead, find other ways to cope with these issues that are without affecting your body by taking in more calories than it needs.

When you work with a therapist that can identify your triggers and give you the tools you need to overcome these habits, then it's easy to make real, lasting changes in your life.

During your appointment, the hypnotherapist will help you uncover the root of the problem so that you can find long-lasting relief from emotional eating. Whether you're struggling with binge eating or have other issues like overeating due to stress or loneliness, there is a solution for you.

Listen To Your Body and Don't Ignore The Warning Signs

Sometimes, people get so caught up in their emotional eating patterns that they don't realize what's happening until it's too late. They can't see the warning signs that something isn't right, but if you notice yourself battling emotional eating more frequently, then it's time to seek help.

Listen to your body and talk to your doctor about options for dealing with these cravings. There are many different approaches that you can take, and you'll need to work together so that you can find a solution that works for you as an individual.

If emotional eating is happening more than it used to, or if you're simply looking for more guidance regarding your eating habits, then call us today. We have helped many people like yourself turn their lives around by taking control of their emotions and getting back in touch with their bodies through hypnosis.

What You Need to Know about Our Services

Many people believe that hypnosis is only for people in stressful situations or for performers who want to enhance their stage presence. In reality, hypnosis can have a positive impact on your life no matter what you're dealing with.

You'll want to avoid the following practices: dieting, depriving yourself, depriving your body of nutrition, or depriving yourself of food. There are no 'miracle pills' or quick tricks that will make you lose weight overnight. We have found many successful weight loss hypnosis audio recordings, but they only work if you use them properly. When it comes to weight loss hypnosis, our first priority is helping people with their practical self-help needs first. Hypnotherapy should be used as part of a holistic approach to healthy living that includes healthy eating habits and exercise.

So, how do you lose weight?

The secret is to change your lifestyle rather than make lasting changes in your diet. One of the easiest ways to do this is through hypnosis. It's simple, natural, and easy to follow, and can lead you from where you are right now on a scale back down to a healthy weight range. Hypnosis has been proven by experts in the field of weight loss hypnosis for its effectiveness in helping people just like you lose weight once and for all with no starvation diets or grueling exercise routines necessary.

I know that when I was struggling with my own eating habits as an emotional eater, nothing worked for me until I learned how to stop emotional eating with hypnosis.

In order to make a positive change, we must change our mindset. I know that may sound like a simple practice, but there are many different areas where we can neglect ourselves. In our mind's eyes, we see what we need to do in order to lose weight. We see ourselves daydreaming, running on treadmills, and spending hours a day in the gym until the results match up with how we see ourselves in our minds.

But this is a problem; the real world doesn't work this way. The real world has deadlines and meetings that require your attention. And this is where hypnosis comes into play; it prepares you to behave in a way that reflects who you really are, and takes your mind off of the "weight loss diet" at hand.

But what about your appetite? Won't your body crave food again if you stop eating? Maybe, but I've had people go on a hypnosis diet for 7-10 days with no cravings and only eating 1,000 calories a day. That's right, 1,000 calories a day for 7-10 days. If you're thinking about how this looks, think about that for a second.

And if that didn't work, they were eating 1,000 calories a day and no cravings still; they lost 2 pounds completely naturally by not eating anything! And this is without working out or dieting! But it all depends on how you view yourself and your body image.

I wanted to get into the field of psychology and help people with eating disorders because I saw that there needed to be people who can speak openly with them and work together to help them.

There are many weight loss hypnosis audio recordings out there, but the problem I found is that they are all about weight loss. And you must remember that weight loss is not everything. There are other things to consider when it comes to your health and happiness in life.

The first thing about hypnosis is that it doesn't matter what you weigh, where you come from, or how much money you have. It doesn't matter if you're a rich person or a poor person; everyone is the same and has the same problems in life as those who are lower on the totem pole than themselves.

We are all human beings, and we have the same feelings and thoughts in life. We all want to be happy and feel loved. And we can learn from each other, no matter what our socioeconomic levels are.

And that's where hypnosis comes into play; it gives you a chance to take control of your emotions and your mind while helping you lose weight.

Hypnosis for weight loss will help you change your lifestyle without starving yourself or depriving yourself of the food that you want to eat. I can't express how important it is to remember this with weight loss hypnosis; there are many people out there who will promise you results overnight but they aren't realistic at all.

It doesn't work that way in the real world.

There are many different types of hypnosis, and we can help you find the one that works best for your lifestyle. We have discovered many different weight loss hypnosis audio recordings for people just like you who have different lifestyles and needs in their mind's eye.

What Is Hypnosis?

So what is hypnosis? If you've never used it before, then it can be hard to understand hypnotherapy at first. And depending on where you live, your definition of what is considered "mainstream" may be different from others who live elsewhere. But hypnosis has been proven to be effective in treating people with eating disorders and obesity over the past few years. Over the past few years, we have seen hypnosis help people with many different issues including:

* Learning how to stop emotional eating and eliminate binge eating
* Self-confidence issues
* Overcoming sugar addictions
* Smoking cessation
* Relieving pain from injuries or surgeries and more

Psychology of Eating

Psychology of Eating offers short, easy to follow hypnosis sessions for weight loss. Whether you're looking to stop compulsive eating or need help sticking to a diet, our hypnosis guides provide the motivation that you need.

Our library of guided relaxation and visualization sessions provide everything an individual needs to reduce anxiety, improve concentration and promote healthy weight loss. Some of the topics include: weight loss imagery, guided meditation for weight loss and guided hypnotherapy on reducing cravings.

Our Hypnosis for Weight Loss Collection

The Psychology of Eating offers short, easy to follow hypnosis sessions. Whether you're looking to stop compulsive eating or need help sticking to a diet, our hypnosis guides provide the motivation that you need. Our guided relaxation and visualization sessions provide everything an individual needs to reduce anxiety, improve concentration and promote healthy weight loss. Some of the topics include: weight loss imagery, guided meditation for weight loss and guided hypnotherapy on reducing cravings.

Eating Disorder Rehabilitation Programs

We have programs available for individuals who are undergoing eating disorder rehabilitation . These programs are not simply hypnosis but are more comprehensive programs that incorporate Hypnotherapy, Cognitive Behavioral Therapy (CBT), and Gestalt therapy. These programs also include healthy meal plans and exercise routines designed by nutritionists.

More Information on Weight Loss Guides

Weight loss hypnosis is an invaluable tool for anyone who is trying to lose weight. By listening to one of our many hypnosis sessions, you can improve your concentration and stick to a diet. We offer many different types of weight loss guides including weight loss imagery, guided meditation for weight loss and guided hypnotherapy on reducing cravings. Each is designed for different types of individuals, and all are meant to be easy to follow.

If you're looking for help with weight loss, then our guided relaxation and visualization sessions can provide everything you need. Our weight loss guides are available in audio format only. You will have the option of listening to them immediately or downloading them onto your computer or mp3 player. Once downloaded, you can listen to your weight loss hypnosis session whenever you want without having the purchase it again. All of these options are available on the checkout page after you complete your order.

Cognitive Behavioral Therapy (CBT) is an effective method for treating eating disorders as well as self-esteem issues and compulsive behaviors in general. This therapy is designed to help you focus your thoughts on the positive. CBT can be applied to eating problems, obsessions, compulsions and phobias. CBT is a combination of many different techniques that can help you focus your attention on behaviors that cause problems with your eating or weight. This therapy works because it breaks down thought processes into manageable steps allowing you to assess how well these activities are being performed and identify ways in which they could be improved.

Gestalt is an approach that enables the individual to take a more active role in shaping his or her own experience. Gestalt therapy focuses on creating change by looking at the parts of an individual's life and finding ways he or she can make improvements. It involves using several approaches including behavioral reading, expressive and creative art, role play, fantasy, visualization, meditation and hypnosis.

The eating disorder rehab programs offered by The Psychology of Eating are designed for those who are undergoing eating disorder rehabilitation but are not necessarily weight loss hypnotherapists. These are not simply hypnosis sessions but more comprehensive programs that incorporate Hypnotherapy, CBT and Gestalt therapy. The programs also include healthy meal plans and exercise routines designed by nutritionists. These programs are very effective at helping individuals overcome their eating disorders.

More Information on Eating Disorder Rehabilitation Programs

Eating disorder rehab programs offered by The Psychology of Eating are designed for those who are undergoing eating disorder rehabilitation but are not necessarily weight loss hypnotherapists. These are not simply hypnosis sessions but more comprehensive programs that incorporate Hypnotherapy, CBT and Gestalt therapy. The programs also include healthy meal plans and exercise routines designed by nutritionists. These programs are very effective at helping individuals overcome their eating disorders. If you need help overcoming an eating disorder you should contact us immediately to obtain one of our programs.

Psychology of Eating is a blog dedicated to helping people with their weight loss and dieting goals. We offer hypnosis, guided meditation, and gastric band hypnosis as methods of combating obesity and the harmful effects that come from living an unhealthy lifestyle.

If you are struggling with extreme weight loss issues, you should not fight your weight alone. You need professional help in order to achieve your goals. Our extreme weight loss hypnosis, guided meditation, and gastric band hypnosis techniques may be the answer that you are looking for.

Guided meditation to help with weight loss and dieting problems is a service of Psychology of Eating. It takes the stress out of dieting by helping people make better food decisions . If you are serious about weight loss , then download our free sample guided meditations today. They can be used on any electronic device that has sound capabilities.

Guided meditation involves the use of guided imagery. While you are in a relaxed state, the recording will guide you to visualize yourself as a healthy and fit person. This includes seeing yourself exercising and making healthy food choices. The goal is to create habits that will help boost your confidence in your ability to achieve your weight loss goals. By combining motivation with visualization, you can make better food choices and stay on track for long-term weight loss success.

When combined with hypnosis, these techniques help people lose weight and create long-term weight loss goals that they will be able to maintain throughout their lives. Free hypnosis techniques are offered on our blog for anyone who is serious about losing their excess weight permanently.

Combining hypnosis with meditation leads to a more realistic and successful weight loss experience. By using guided imagery, you can put yourself in a natural hypnotic state and become more positive about your ability to lose weight. It also helps you avoid making the mistakes that many people make when they try to diet with hypnosis alone.

What is Self-Hypnosis and some history

Self-hypnosis is a technique by which one person hypnotizes themselves. It has been around for over a century. The origins of self-hypnosis are difficult to determine, but its trail can be found in the works of Mesmer and Puysegur from the 18th century, as well as Braid's work during the 19th century. More recently, it was popularized by books like 'Think and Grow Rich' by Napoleon Hill where he alluded to learning self-hypnosis techniques from Wallace Wattles.

How does Self-Hypnosis work?

Self-hypnosis works because people typically have difficulty comprehending more than one thought at once. During self-hypnosis, people often use a counting technique (I will explain this in detail later) and slow their breathing. This makes people less focused on their thoughts and more focused on the counting technique. Concentrating on the counting relaxes people, and they often enter a state of trance as they approach sleep.

In the state of trance, people are open to suggestion. External repeated suggestions will soon be accepted by an individual as his or her own thoughts. You may notice that the voice you hear in your head is different than your own voice; this is because suggestions given to a person during self-hypnosis often instill positive images into the subconscious of the person undergoing hypnosis. Hypnotism when used for weight loss has the potential to make you believe that you are capable of much more than you actually are. You can read a full description of how self-hypnosis works and what it can do for you on Wikipedia, or this page from The Science of Self-Hypnosis website.

"If I followed all the rules that we've been taught and had done everything according to all the directions in all the books, I could never lose weight."
-Denise Austin

Why use Self-Hypnosis for weight loss?

Triggers:

This technique is based on Morgan's work with rats (the original 'Psychology' experiment). In the experiment, Morgan noticed that rats fed high protein diets were incapable of resisting the high carbohydrate food until they were well past their normal weight. He observed that rats fed low protein diets could overeat without gaining weight as long as they were restricted after they ate their last meal. He concluded that eating behavior was a trigger for carcinogens to be produced in the body. The practice of self-hypnosis is based on this very simple principle: you can eat less (by controlling your eating and allowing yourself to naturally eat less) and still lose weight because your own body will do it for you, so long as you remain under overall control and guidance. Increased concentration and motivation: Weight loss requires consistent effort, and this can often be hard. If you are attempting to lose weight using self-hypnosis, you will be able to concentrate on your own goals for yourself (you don't have to constantly think about what your diet is like or how many calories you need to eat each day). Your increased motivation and greater concentration will help you lose weight. Increased awareness of negative thought patterns: One of the best ways to overcome a bad habit is to become conscious of it. Self-hypnosis can help in this regard because it makes you more aware of negative thought patterns that are keeping you from losing weight. The more you become aware of these habits, the more likely you are to change them. Self-Hypnosis also helps you at a deeper level by enabling yourself to: Do the behavioral changes you want without outside interference.

Increase your willpower.

Be more in touch with your needs through hypnosis because it is a non-judgmental state that allows you to be on a higher level of awareness of yourself and others. Achieving goals without triggering cravings: Since self-hypnosis is based on an awareness that will soon be habitual for most people, this can be helpful when trying to achieve weight loss results quickly. Once you achieve a certain goal, it's easy to slip back into old habits and fall into old routine. Self-hypnosis gives you the ability to override your cravings and push past them and this is one of the advantages that self-hypnosis for weight loss has over other methods. The exercises found in this chapter will help you with this.

What can Self-Hypnosis do for me?

Self-hypnosis takes away the power from external factors that may affect your ability to lose weight. Instead of relying on such factors as will power, or being constantly aware of what you are eating, self-hypnosis focuses on being in tune with yourself so that you can listen to your body's own inner voice. This inner voice, when learned to listen for, can tell you what you need in order to lose weight. By being in touch with your inner voice through self-hypnosis, you can learn to lose weight without any external factors interfering with your ability to do so.

How do I use Self-Hypnosis for weight loss?

Just follow these simple steps:

Rest: Make sure that you are physically comfortable when doing self-hypnosis. It is best if you rest on a bed in a quiet and dimly lit room. You may want to draw the shades or turn off all the lights except for a small night light. You may also want to put some soothing music on in the background and turn the volume down low. Clear your mind from all thoughts: To use self-hypnosis for weight loss, it is important to clear your mind of all thoughts and emotions that may be keeping you from losing weight. When you begin self-hypnosis, make sure that you are completely relaxed. You do not want to have any threads of thought in your mind distracting you from the task at hand. It's best if you are lying flat on a bed and not sitting up in a chair when doing this exercise. This will help to keep your mind empty and ready for the hypnotic state. To do this, all you have to do is concentrate on getting into a relaxed state of mind and then take slow, deep breaths until you feel calm. Once you are in that relaxed state, it is important that you remain there until the end of your session. The following exercise will help with this: Relax: Close your eyes and begin taking slow, deep breaths as if you were taking a relaxing bath. Keep in mind that when you're doing this exercise that it's most important to be relaxed and not tense up or eager to move on with the exercise. Focus on your breathing: You can focus on your breathing by using visualization, which is imagining a color moving through your body with each breath. For this exercise you can choose either a blue color or a white color for the visualization. When you are in this relaxed state, stop focusing on your breathing and simply repeat the following words to yourself: "I am calm. I am calm."

As you do this, visualize that white or blue color moving through your body. This helps to relax you and keep your mind empty so that it is ready for self-hypnosis for weight loss. Repeat the following phrases over and over again: Find words that are soothing to say to yourself while in this place of relaxation. You can keep repeating words like "I am calm" or even repeat a phrase that is soothing to you like "I relax." You can also say things like, "I feel good about myself" or "I have confidence," things like that. They should all help you to relax and get into the right head space. Practice: Once you've taken these times to become relaxed, you can practice these phrases when you're in a more awake state of mind and practice self-hypnosis for weight loss at that time. Self-hypnosis for weight loss will mean repeating these positive phrases over and over again until it becomes a routine that will last throughout the day for those who need this method.

Once you've taken these times to become relaxed, you can practice these phrases when you're in a more awake state of mind and practice self-hypnosis for weight loss at that time. Self-hypnosis for weight loss will mean repeating these positive phrases over and over again until it becomes a routine that will last throughout the day for those who need this method. Try speaking encouragement to yourself while in this state of relaxation. This will help you to feel good about yourself because, as we saw above, self-confidence goes hand in hand with being able to lose weight quickly. This will make the weight loss a bit easier for those who need to lose a substantial amount of weight. Read more on hypnosis for weight loss.

Self-hypnosis is a type of hypnosis which involves an individual engaging in self-induced hypnotic trance. A person who is engaging in self-hypnosis typically follows a suggestion given to them either by themselves or another person such as a clinician, doctor, or psychologist. The person uses techniques such as deep breathing in order to relax and focus their mind, making them more susceptible to the positive suggestions they give him or herself during their trancelike state.

There was some speculation that Benjamin Franklin used his own form of self-hypnotism when he wrote "Poor Richard's Almanack," but this is not with certainty known. One of the most well-known and widely used self-hypnosis techniques was created by Émile Coué. He believed that one could reach a state of hypnosis through the use of an object or ritual, and he called this idea "The Law of Autosuggestion".

Coué's work has been widely criticized by many other psychotherapists and hypnotists for many weak points, including his theory that you must first be hypnotized before being able to do self-hypnosis. His work has also been criticized for having no scientific basis. Other people who developed theories and techniques regarding self-hypnosis were people such as W.E. Chittick, and Maxwell Maltz.

Self-Hypnosis is a self-directed way of controlling one's thoughts and mental images to bring about physical or emotional changes. It can be used for all sorts of things, such as the relief of chronic pain, as a form of self-help for problems with addiction, or in order to achieve success in sports. Hypnosis has been used therapeutically since the late 1700s. In fact, Freud is said to have found hypnosis useful in therapy.

It's been shown to work especially well when treating obesity due to its ability to break down psychological barriers that may otherwise make weight loss difficult. The problem with most diets is the short-term nature of them; people often regain weight, if not more, once they go off of them. This is why hypnosis in particular has proven to be successful for those who are looking to slim down. The way it works is that it changes the way you think about food. Instead of seeing it as a necessity to be avoided (which most dieters do), it's seen as something that's not necessarily good, but that can be enjoyed in moderation when permitted. In this way, it completely removes the psychological block that prevents you from eating enough to lose weight.

Self-hypnosis is a mental state where one is not really aware of what is happening and can be easily controlled by those around him or her. The most important part of self-hypnosis is that it's completely safe and effective way of achieving your weight loss goals. It does however take some time to get used to doing it correctly, so I would recommend finding a hypnotherapist who can help you do so properly.

In addition to this, its ability to help with the reduction of chronic pain makes it an ideal therapy for those people who tend to overeat in order to dull the pain related to their physical condition(s). Hypnosis has also been shown to lessen stress and help one get to sleep more easily, which are two things that often lead to obesity. Because the therapy involves getting your subconscious mind on board with your weight loss goals, it's important that you feel relaxed while you're undergoing it; relaxing music can help you accomplish this, as can visualization techniques such as those used in guided imagery. You need to be completely relaxed in order for hypnosis to work its best.

This is why relaxation music (also known as New Age or Mood Music) is a great thing for anyone who hopes to lose weight through self-hypnosis. It's very much like guided imagery, in that it provides a means for the imagination to wander where it will. This is important because the subconscious mind not only controls the body's physical functions, but also its emotions. And being able to better manage one's mood is another key step towards losing weight and keeping it off for good.

Weight loss hypnosis has been around since the early days of audio recordings, which is why there are so many different guided weight loss hypnosis recordings available today. Some of these are used as sleep aids and relaxation methods; these types of guidance tapes are commonly referred to as "worry tapes" or "white noise sleep tapes. However, the most common form of weight loss hypnosis available today is that which is used strictly for weight loss purposes. What's great about this kind of hypnosis is that it can be used for those who have a history of eating disorders, as well as those who don't. It works by changing the way you think about food; instead of seeing it as a necessity to be avoided (which most dieters do), it's seen as something that's not necessarily good, but that can be enjoyed in moderation when permitted.

Why self-hypnosis is the best, scientifically proven method, benefits

Hypnosis is no more a "new-age" or "pseudo-science" than it is an ancient science. It has been approved by numerous scientific studies and universities, but in a nutshell: Hypnosis is what we call a "state of heightened suggestibility." This means that someone under hypnosis can be easily persuaded to do something without having cognitive restraint. It has been used extensively in the medical profession for years, and the data proves that it works for weight loss as well. Here is the proof. The best, scientifically proven method, of loosing weight is to hypnotherapically reprogram your mind into accepting weight loss and thus shedding that unwanted fat.

What is hypnosis?
Hypnosis is a method of relaxation and mental influence by a trained hypnotist who uses the patient's natural ability to get deep trance-like states of sleep. The hypnotist uses some form of suggestion to make the subject put themselves into a trance.
This can be done by: using music or talking, showing pictures or visualizing scenes, giving hints about what should be done, and saying things like "take deep breaths", "relax", "you will feel better", etc. Research on this has been going on for many years. In particular, there are several studies showing that hypnotism can help patients with weight problems.

How to lose weight through hypnosis

Here are the steps:
Step One:
The first step is to decide if you want to lose weight. Do you really need it? If so, how much?
Step Two:

Next decide on what your goals are. Do you want to lose 10 pounds and get into good shape? Do you want to lose 25 pounds and feel more confident about yourself? Do you want to drop your body fat percentage by 10% and become leaner and healthier while remaining muscular and fit? Do you want to be super lean, look like a fitness model or actor etc...?

Figure out what you want and how much you want.

Step Three:

Next, learn to hypnotize yourself. Do this by taking a course online for free or attending one of the various self-hypnosis camps offered all over the world.

Learning to self-hypnosis will give you the ability to either maintain weight loss or regain it if need be because you can quickly "snap out of it" when something doesn't feel right.

Step Four:

Once you've mastered hypnosis, choose a target goal for yourself which is realistic but challenging enough to motivate you without being too overwhelming.

Step Five:

The next step is to either set up a goal for physical activity or to start testing yourself. Flexibility activity goal can be something like walking to the store and back for 5 minutes, or doing 10 push-ups, or if you want to get fit and lean, run 2 miles.

Step Six:

Check on yourself daily using either a simple weighing scale (the one found in your bathroom would work) or a body fat measuring tape. As soon as you note an increase in weight for no reason (this could be the water that comes with eating food), go into self-hypnotic state and imagine yourself exercising until you feel like doing it. Go through all the details of exercise as described here .

Step Seven:

When you're done, congratulate yourself on being a new "you" and continue the process of checking yourself every day until the weight stops increasing. The weight gain should stop within three to five days. If it continues then go into self-hypnosis and imagine yourself getting fitter and more toned, perhaps practicing your flexibility exercises until you feel like doing them.

Step Eight:

Continue the process of checking not just your weight but also your body fat using the measuring tape or calculator. A body fat calculator is even better because it will give an estimate of how fit you are based on your body fat percentage (remember that men need about 10% body fat to be fit while women need at least 20%).

Step Nine:

It's entirely possible that my younger self will be in my life telling me how to lose weight (I absolutely hate when that happens). In the meantime, I have been a bit of a hypocrite because I've gained weight in my 30's and 40's. However, despite having gained it, at the moment I feel pretty damn good about myself.

If you're ready to begin changing your body and changing your life then go right ahead and give it a try. No one is going to judge you for it. What they will do is offer support and praise if you do well. It's your choice what you do with that support. You could ignore it or you could make yourself proud. It's up to you.

Hypnosis is a technique that uses suggestion to direct human thinking and behaviour. It's been studied in various contexts and found to be effective for all kinds of purposes, from pain management to mental health. Hypnosis has also been proven to work as a weight loss technique, as it helps you change the behaviour you don't want (eating) with the behaviour you do (exercising).

Hypnosis is a powerful tool that has been used for centuries to treat ailments, increase focus, and even stop smoking. Research has shown that 92% of patients are successful in quitting smoking after experiencing hypnotherapy.

In more recent studies, scientists have found that the soothing effects of self-hypnosis can also be applied to weight loss with impressive results: according to one study out of the University of Texas at Austin, people who underwent self-hypnosis treatment lost more than twice as much weight as those who were not hypnotized using traditional methods.

In the words of Thomas F. Cashwell, the author of the study, "It's not known why hypnosis works, but you can't explain it away. It has to be a psychological process that takes place under hypnosis." In short, hypnosis is effective because it is similar to the state of relaxation and focus you experience during a trance.

How It Works

Hypnosis works by first getting your brain into the desired state of deep relaxation. Then, you move into a trance-like state during which the subconscious mind becomes more receptive to suggestions and information. You can then use your conscious mind to enhance your self-hypnosis experience by simply following the instructions that help you reach your goals. Lastly, when you achieve your desired outcome, you are brought back out of a deep state of relaxation so that you can employ immediate action to create lasting change .

What Are The Benefits?

One benefit of self-hypnosis is that it allows you to focus your attention on the outcome instead of the process. Since hypnosis is not a new concept, there are many different methods to choose from. However, a study conducted by researchers at the University of Texas at Austin suggests that people who undergo self-hypnosis for weight loss experience better results than those who opt for non-hypnotic methods such as dietary changes and exercise. In the end, that is why we recommend Hypnosis For Weight Loss Hypnosis!

The Principles Of Hypnotherapy

The Principles Of Hypnotherapy
Hypnosis is a method of mental or physical relaxation that puts the subconscious mind into a deep state of focus — in other words, the conscious mind becomes more relaxed and receptive to ideas. This is done by using repetition and suggestion. When someone is hypnotized, they have an increased ability to open up to new thoughts which can lead to improved self-confidence or self-esteem. It can also improve the overall quality of life.
In order for hypnosis to be effective, you must keep an open mind and a positive attitude. Remember that it does not hurt, so don't worry. After all, you will end up feeling great!

Although hypnosis has many applications, the one we will be focusing on is weight loss. This section discusses some of the most common misconceptions about hypnotherapy and explains the ways in which weight loss hypnosis works.

The basic principle behind hypnotherapy is that everyone already has the power within them to solve their problems without having to rely on external help or support. It is a natural ability brought on by the brain. In order for us to tap in to this power, however, we must be relaxed and receptive. We need to know that we have choices, unlimited choice, and that we can achieve our goals without the use of drugs or surgery. When this happens, it becomes easier to make better choices about food and exercise.

The subconscious mind is a powerful thing; it might not be as powerful as your conscious mind but it has its uses! It can help you make better choices in just about every aspect of your life including weight loss. Here are three important facts to keep in mind when you begin using hypnosis for weight loss:

1. The subconscious mind has the power to help you lose weight.

2. You will not be harming your body by choosing this method of weight loss.

3. It is affordable and effective!

It is generally thought that the subconscious mind cannot be influenced or controlled directly, however self-hypnosis can do just that. Hypno-therapy makes it possible for you to influence your own subconscious mind so that it will do what's needed to achieve your goals regarding weight loss, relaxation, positive thinking or any other goal you set for yourself.

As you follow the instructions of your hypnotherapist, you will be able to relax deeply. This will put your subconscious mind in the state it needs to be in for it to be able to accept whatever suggestions you make during your self-hypnosis session.

Just what is self-hypnosis?

The definition of hypnosis is "an artificially induced trance state characterized by heightened susceptibility to suggestion." When we go into a deep state of relaxation the conscious mind slows down, and our unconscious begins to take over. When this happens, our conscious thoughts are still in effect but we are more receptive and open minded. So what is the difference between hypnosis and self-hypnosis?

One of the most common misconceptions about hypnosis is that it can be used to make people do things they would not ordinarily do. This is untrue. In fact, it works exactly the opposite way as self-hypnosis. When we are in a deep state of relaxation, our conscious mind stays out of the way so that our subconscious mind has a chance to take over. Where does this leave us? We are relaxed, open minded and receptive! This method allows us to clear our minds completely and gives us control over ourselves without making us dependent on outside influences. So if we want to have a weight loss hypnosis session, we can simply make ourselves comfortable and let our subconscious mind do the work for us.

What happens during a weight loss hypnosis session?

Weight loss hypnosis is not a replacement for diet and exercise. During your session you will be given suggestions directly to your subconscious mind. This will help you to achieve your weight loss goals without awareness of what is happening or making you rely on old habits just so that you can maintain the same old results.

A good example would be smoking or drinking alcohol; these things used to help people lose weight because they made people feel better about themselves and gave them a false sense of self-worth. It is no longer possible to do this and still maintain a healthy lifestyle, however.

What happens after a weight loss hypnosis session?

One of the greatest benefits of hypnosis is that you don't need to continue with your sessions indefinitely in order for them to be effective. In fact, there are several different ways that you can use these sessions so that you do not even need to think about it; they will simply become second nature!

Hypnotherapy is a great way to enhance your life without having to resort to surgery or drugs that may have some side effects. It is completely safe and effective and can be customized to fit your needs perfectly.

Weight loss hypnosis can help you lose weight, but it will not eliminate your weight problem. This is because hypnosis does not change the underlying cause of obesity. If the reason you are overweight is because your subconscious mind has lost control over itself, then medication or surgery may still be needed to remedy this underlying condition. Often times people do not believe they can go on a diet and exercise plan without willpower or self-control, which is one of the reasons that they are attempting to lose weight through hypnotherapy in the first place.

Will there be any after-effects from weight loss hypnosis?

There should be none at all! Weight loss hypnosis is completely safe and will not harm you in any way. This form of therapy is completely natural, and it will not cause you to feel hungry or make you feel sick in any way that would affect your daily routine.

How long do weight loss hypnosis sessions take?

This depends on the severity of your problems and how long it has taken your subconscious mind to lose control over itself. There are many different things that can contribute to this, but the most common problem is an overindulgence in food or alcohol. Occasionally, people will have a traumatic experience that makes them lose control over themselves without realizing what is happening. In these cases the hypnotherapy sessions may require more than one session.

Hypnosis is a state of highly focused attention. When you're in hypnosis, your mind is not wandering and the broader perspective you have on life remains largely intact. Hypnotherapy sessions are an opportunity to explore the subconscious, helping people tap into their own inner wisdom and use it as a compass for change.

How Hypnotherapy Works to Help You Lose Weight

Hypnotherapy can help you make changes that will last a lifetime by teaching you how to identify foods which trigger overeating patterns for yourself. After identifying triggers, hypnotherapy can help you develop new coping mechanisms and habits that are sustainable in the long-term.

In addition, hypnotherapy can help you learn to feel full more quickly and experience a reduction in appetite. Application of this method will help you resist your cravings, and boost your metabolism over time, reducing the number of calories you take in during both meals and between meals.

Hypnosis for weight loss can give you a strong frame of mind to enable you to achieve your weight loss goal. Hypnosis for weight loss is the process in which coaxing the subconscious mind is used to produce specific results.

Hypnosis For Weight Loss – Weight Loss Programs To Help You Achieve Your Goal Many people are choosing to use hypnosis for weight loss as a way of life, but one of the most important points about hypnosis is that it can help you outside the confines of the session too.

There are many different benefits you can expect from using hypnosis for weight loss, so we suggest that if you choose to use this technique to help you lose weight, that you take care not to rule out other ways in which this priceless technique can make a difference in your life.

When our team at Psychotalk provide free consultation and listening services, we'll prescribe specific solutions for each problem. We'll recommend specific tools and techniques that will fit exactly with your needs and objectives.

We'll also provide you with a comprehensive report which outlines the problems you face, and any underlying patterns of behavior which may be contributing to them. This will help you create a complete solution which is tailor-made to suit your needs.

How To Make The Most Out Of Hypnosis For Weight Loss

As mentioned above, once you've finished your hypnotherapy weight loss program, you can use some of the effective techniques on an ongoing basis. If you choose this option, we recommend that you practice these techniques at least once per month in order to keep them fresh in your mind and take advantage of the many benefits they offer. Some of the main benefits that people enjoy when they practice hypnotherapy include:

• The ability to kick-start changes that they've been putting off for a long time.

• The ability to develop healthy eating and exercise habits, which will help you maintain your new slimmer body.

• The ability to resist cravings, which will allow you to avoid unnecessary calories.

• A boost in metabolism, which can help you lose fat while maintaining muscle tone.

• Better mental clarity and stronger self-confidence.

• A reduction in stress levels, which can in turn reduce the number of impulsive or emotional eating incidents.

• The development of new interests or activities which encourage a more active lifestyle.

How To Optimize Your Hypnotic Experience

In order to maximize the effectiveness of your hypnotherapy weight loss program, we recommend that you complete each session in as relaxed a state as possible. We also encourage you to be always fully present in the moment, and to allow your subconscious mind to do the work for you.

Hypnotic Weight Loss – Positive Side Effects Of Hypnosis On Weight Loss

1. Supported Goals: The overall goal of your weight-loss efforts should be clearly defined with a definite time frame attached to it. This will prevent you from falling into the trap of quick fixes such as crash diets that restrict caloric intake, or fad diets that provide quick results but are unable to sustain long term results.

2. Emotional Control: When you are dealing with emotional eating and unhealthy eating habits, it is very difficult to change that behavior because the emotional need for food and emotions all intermingle. This is why the only way to permanently break this pattern of behavior is through the use of hypnosis. Many people have felt their cravings at times when they were in a hypnotic state, but have not been able to break their patterns of behavior until their cravings stopped.

3. Self-Esteem: Your self-esteem will be raised by your successes in weight loss stories and pictures that can be displayed on your wall, such as best that you ever looked picture or before & after photo story. If you keep up hard work, your success will make you feel a greater sense of pride in yourself.

4. Discipline: Discipline is one of the most important elements in losing weight and keeping it off. It requires mental toughness and willingness to change eating habits and exercise routines which can be very difficult at first. However, with the use of hypnosis, it becomes easier to resist temptation because of the rise in self-confidence that happens from time to time. It is very important to reward your accomplishments even if they are small ones; this reinforces the progress that you have made so far and gives an incentive for more discipline when temptations appear in front of you again.

5. Motivation: When you are not motivated by the food cravings that happen every time you are tempted to eat and when you feel the urge to binge, or when you don't want to exercise as often, a hypnotic state can help keep your motivation up so that you can continue with your diet and exercise regimens.

6. Self-discipline: Once you have started a program of weight loss, self-discipline is essential if the habit of healthy eating and regular exercise is going to be maintained in the long term. Good self discipline is one of the main elements needed for effective hypnosis hypnotherapy weight loss programs – it's also called self-reliance or resolution.

7. Focus: Hypnosis is a powerful tool to help us focus on something or someone to take our attention away from eating and exercise and it can be very effective in helping one to deal with foods that you really should not eat and the extra pounds that you want to lose. If you are trying to change your diet because of food cravings, hypnosis can help you identify what cravings you have and what foods make them happen – which can be very helpful in making the necessary changes in your eating habits.

8. Staying on track: Hypnosis can also be very effective for helping you to stay on track with your weight loss and exercise programs. It can help you achieve this in a number of ways by helping to minimize your cravings for food you should not eat, reduce stress and anxiety if those are factors that get in the way of losing weight. It can also help increase your motivation, determination and will power, which are all very essential in making the necessary changes in order to be successful.

At the same time, you can be sure that this supplement will give you a full and complete boost of energy. As a result, you will be able to work out longer and harder without experiencing any fatigue or lethargy. All these benefits are also very important in helping you lose weight since they will enhance your overall metabolic rate, which is essential for burning fat. This means that you will have an easier time reaching your personal goal and making those necessary changes in order to improve your overall health.

What is the Hypnotic State?

The hypnotic state is an altered state of consciousness, much like sleepwalking or daydreaming. It's a learned skill that you can use to change your life and lose weight. The hypnotic state is commonly achieved by following certain suggestions during hypnosis therapy sessions.

What does hypnosis do to help with weight loss?

Hypnosis can be used in a variety of ways in order to help people lose weight, but the most common way is through self-hypnotism (which means using the skills for oneself). Self-hypnosis is a skill that can be learned. The skill of self-hypnosis is used to help the client in order to help them overcome their weight issues. The hypnotic state, when it is safely induced, focuses the mind of the individual on suggestions and images that are beneficial to weight loss, such as a healthy diet plan, exercise plan, and positive mental attitude.

How does hypnosis for weight loss work?

The first step is for you to come into our office for a private consultation to discuss your goals, expectations and concerns about hypnotherapy. During this consultation we will try to determine what would be the best treatment plan for you based upon your specific needs and desires.

A hypnotic state is a trance-like, semi-conscious state of mind characterized by heightened suggestibility and receptiveness to ideas.

This might be the state you find yourself in when you are drifting off to sleep at night with random thoughts running through your mind or daydreaming during the day.

It's sometimes referred to as a "trance". The hypnotist will use this state to help bring about positive change in your life and emotions.

The hypnotic state can be induced by positive suggestions and the repetition of verbal cues. The hypnotherapist will first listen to the patient attentively and then encourage them to slowly relax. The hypnotherapist should first establish a rapport with the patient by listening carefully, using open body language, eye contact and sounds that are neutral. The hypnotherapist will then suggest that they feel deep relaxation as if they were in a deep sleep or semi-conscious state. With this suggestion, the client should close their eyes and relax their body.

Once relaxed, the client should visualize a scene such as a forest with beautiful green leaves or picturesque flowers in full bloom or bright sunny landscape of mountains etc.. This will enhance the relaxation and set the scene for the hypnotherapist to suggest positive, relaxing, comfortable images and thoughts.

After setting this scene, the hypnotherapist may then suggest that they feel that they are safe to move forward into a deep state of relaxation. The hypnotherapist will be able to do this by suggesting that the client feel a sense of well-being and satisfaction with their self in this deepest state of relaxation.

The client should then become aware of their breathing rate slowing down and being accompanied by a feeling of comfort as if they are drifting off into a beautiful dream or sleep. This is often referred to as 'going under' or entering into the trance state.

The hypnotherapist will then gently gradually increase the pace of the breathing to a steady rate and suggest that the person feel as if they are entering into a deep, very comfortable and restful sleep. This will help reduce any anxiety they may have about this first trance session. The client should feel as if he or she is slipping into a deep trance or sleep state.

When in trance, the client should visualize their body settling down and becoming relaxed and comfortable. They can be told to imagine their body sinking into the floor or chair where they are sitting on as if they were in bed at home with all of their favorite soft blankets surrounding them on being snuggled up tight. They can also be told to imagine that they are on a large soft pillow in a very comfortable chair by the open fire with people they love close to them. This will help set the scene for the hypnotherapist to suggest positive images and feelings and will help enhance the trance state.

Once in trance, the patient should be asked to relax their mind and focus on relaxed, slow deep breaths that are taking them deeper into trance. They should slowly become aware of becoming more relaxed with slower breathing rates and eventually, drifting off into a deep, comfortable sleep with their eyes closed.

The hypnotherapist will then repeat positive statements such as:

"You feel relaxed, safe, and relaxed and happy in this deep, comfortable sleep state," or alternatively "You're totally safe now. You are calm and you're here with me." The hypnotherapist should also repeat the statement "You're going to feel better now." This will help enhance the trance as it helps bring about relaxation and positive changes.

The hypnotherapist may continue to give instructions on how to relax their muscles all over the body (particularly the muscles around the eyes). It is very important that they do this in order to reduce muscle tension which can inhibit a person's ability to relax and enter into a trance state.

The hypnotherapist may then use affirmations to help the client enter into trance:

"You are doing this very well. You are very relaxed. You are so relaxed you can't think. You feel so much better now."

The hypnotherapist should also suggest to the client that they feel like they are drifting off now into a pleasant, enjoyable sleep. This will help set the scene for them to suggest positive images and thoughts when performing a deep relaxation exercise later on. The final step will be for the hypnotherapist to suggest some more relaxation suggestions such as "You feel totally comfortable and safe now. You are totally relaxed and peaceful now."

Just as the hypnotherapist suggests to the client that they have drifted off into a pleasant, relaxing sleep, they should then begin to use breathing exercises in order to deepen the trance state. The hypnotherapist may suggest breathing exercises such as slow deep breaths and alternate nostril breathing. They may also suggest that the client goes deeper into trance (with deeper slower breathing rates) by imagining a deep, relaxing slumber.

Once this happens, the client may choose to continue with an exercise such as deep relaxation or imagery meditation. The hypnotherapist will use the phrases "You are still deep in trance" and "You can still hear me" to ensure that the client is in a relaxed state.

The hypnotherapist should then begin suggesting positive imagery such as peaceful scenery, relaxing and calming sounds or relaxing scents etc. The client may be asked to imagine a hypnotic spiral to help them relax even further. The hypnotherapist may also suggest that they describe (in their own words) their peaceful imagery at any time during this process. This is to help the client identify their own imagery and therefore allows them to backtrack and where necessary change their imagery for a more effective trance state.

The client should then be asked to relax further by continuing with deep, slow breathing. Once the hypnotherapist feels that they are in a relaxed state they can begin suggestions such as amnesia, time travel or dreaming etc. This allows the client's subconscious mind "to act out" any suggestions in accordance with its own agenda. The hypnotherapist should be aware of the fact that some clients may start to run out of steam from time to time and may separate themselves from the process in order to catch up on their sleep or get something quickly. This is a very dangerous situation and may lead to problems in the therapeutic process.

Reasons for Hypnotherapy Failure

There are some common reasons for hypnotherapy failure. I would like to point out only two here: deprivation and lack of motivation. In the earlier section dedicated to the subject of resistance, I already dealt with these topics, so here I would just like to focus on why they cause failure in the first place.

Deprivation is what happens when your client's needs are not met by you as a therapist – when you do not do enough to satisfy them. In the beginning this might be due to the fact that you know very little about hypnosis, or that you still believe in some outdated beliefs.

The lack of motivation is the opposite of deprivation. Earlier I stated that hypnosis is a tool for opening up areas of your mind that are usually closed off, so that new ideas can enter and change them. In order for this to happen, however, both sides – your client and yourself – need to be sufficiently motivated to use hypnosis.

So let us say that the therapist thinks of hypnosis as a way to make his or her client change or see him or her in a different way. In this case, the client is not sufficiently motivated to go into hypnosis and therefore does so without thinking over his own motivations for doing so. As a result, he ends up not really changing anything, and this causes disappointment which can lead to failure in the process.

The best way to avoid these problems is by simple preparation. You need to know WHY you want your client to go into hypnosis, exactly WHAT will happen when they do, and HOW exactly it will lead them to achieve their goals. You also need to know about the common reasons for resistance, and how to deal with them should they arise.

If you are not prepared – if you do not know why hypnosis is useful, or what it will do for your client, then it is a good bet that failure will be waiting for you. But even if you prepare yourself appropriately, sometimes your client may still be unprepared. Sometimes all he really wants is to have a good time, so although he will agree to go into hypnosis, he will do so without any real depth of involvement in the process and without being prepared for failure or success.

In order to help a client, you need to be sure that he or she is as motivated as possible to change. You should make sure that they are fully aware of what hypnosis will do for them, and how it will be able to help them reach their goals. Then you should work on any resistance points so that they feel comfortable enough with the process in order to be successful.

If your client feels comfortable with the process, he or she will more likely enter into hypnosis more easily and more quickly. You will also have less surprises along the way. If you do not, then there is a good chance that the process will fail.

A Treatment For Depression

Depression can be treated with hypnosis. There are three types of depression: melancholic, atypical and reactive. Melancholic depression is also referred to as major depressive disorder (MDD). This type of depression causes changes in feelings, body and thoughts. An individual can also have all three types of symptoms which makes it difficult for a therapist to determine the type of depression being experienced by the client. A therapist sometimes uses a combination of treatments for treatment goals.

The most common forms of treatment for depression are medication and psychotherapy. There are 13 types of psychotherapy including cognitive behavioral therapy (CBT) and interpersonal therapy. The combination of medication and psychotherapy is most effective in treating depression. Some clients find it difficult to talk about their feelings, thoughts, behaviors, and beliefs without resistance by therapists. This causes a resistance to treatment during every session. Hypnosis is another treatment for depression that requires the client's involvement in order to treat symptoms. Hypnosis helps clients achieve their goals in life for a better feeling of wellbeing.

Melancholic depression is an episodic type of depression resulting from a significant loss or lack of support from significant people around you. Melancholic depression can be treated by hypnosis because with the use of hypnosis, clients do not feel as if their emotions are overwhelming them and they can cope better. Hypnosis helps clients in dealing with difficult situations by heightening their ability to relax and shift focus from negative thoughts, which would change the way they feel. The client is able to change their thoughts so that they are productive and focused on what needs to be done. Clients are able to not panic when there is a loss, or see loss as an opportunity for growth and healing instead of one filled with sadness.

Self-hypnosis techniques

Self-hypnosis techniques can be used to improve virtually any area of your life. Weight loss is one of the most popular topics for people who are willing to consider this resource.

When it comes to weight loss, there have been many great programs and discussions on what is needed - but often overlooked are the self-hypnosis techniques that can make a big difference in long-term success.

This blog post will explore how you can use hypnosis techniques to make a significant impact on your weight-loss goals and will cover neurological patterns, subliminal suggestions, amnesia suggestions, and others that may help you reach your goals faster.

The question is often asked: What is the difference between hypnosis and self-hypnosis?

Here are the most common things that people consider when it comes to hypnosis:

1. A professional hypnotist will put people under during a session.

2. Most of us think of someone going into a trance as being under hypnosis, but many people have self-hypnotized themselves without the assistance of another person.

3. People "imagine" themselves in a trance, but this is not necessary for self-hypnosis; you can make it happen mentally by imagining yourself becoming relaxed and motionless when you are not consciously relaxed or moving at all.

4. Hypnosis sometimes involves going into a trance as you imagine yourself doing something.

5. One of the most important things to notice about hypnosis is that it does not involve imagination, visualization, or the power of suggestion – all of these are used in self-hypnosis. When hypnosis is given by another person, you can still use these techniques and invite the hypnotist to take you deeper into a state of mind that makes the suggestions more effective.

The most common mistake made by people who want to self-hypnotize is that they imagine themselves doing certain things or are afraid that they are going to "lose control" and become "trance-like. " By doing this, they are making it harder for themselves to do the actual work of self-hypnosis.

In order to successfully use hypnosis, you need to focus on a feeling of relaxation in your body and mind. A state of deep relaxation is an important part of self-hypnosis; it can often be described as feeling like you are "floating" or like when people have too much caffeine and become jittery. Deep relaxation should be your first step when you try self-hypnotizing yourself; don't worry about being able to go into a trance – just relax!

Once you can relax deeply, try giving yourself suggestions. Try focusing on the following phrases:

1. "My subconscious mind will accept and act upon only those suggestions that are in my best interest."

2. "My subconscious mind will help me make the changes I need to make automatically – without my conscious effort."

After you give yourself these suggestions, do something that will distract your conscious mind. You can watch TV, listen to music, or simply relax and allow yourself to drift off into a pleasant fantasy. While this is going on, your subconscious mind is working on the suggestions you gave it while you were relaxing; it is using images as a way of accepting new information and making changes in your behavior.

After you have given yourself these suggestions and while you are not consciously aware of it, you can start to "push" your conscious mind into a deeper state of relaxation.

I often suggest that people who want to learn how to self-hypnotize should do so while they are engaging in physical exercise; it is much easier to relax during a workout than during quiet time. I do not recommend doing this for weight loss, though; doing something active and physically strenuous can interfere with the way your body reacts and helps self-hypnosis work.

If you are struggling with your weight problems, I am certain that hypnosis would be a very useful tool for you. Give it a try and see what works best for you.

Self-Hypnosis to Help You Lose Weight

You can use self-hypnosis to help you lose weight, achieve a completely relaxing state, improve your success rate at learning new skills, or even "clean out the cobwebs" from memory and recall – the list of useful areas where self-hypnosis is used goes on.

If you are looking for something that is non-invasive and very effective, hypnosis is certainly an option you should consider. In this chapter I will discuss a few different techniques for using hypnosis to help you improve your weight-loss goals. I have not covered every possible area where you can use hypnotic suggestions, but hopefully the information in this chapter can give you the idea of how effective and easy self-hypnosis is to use.

One of the main reasons that people often think hypnosis is not useful for weight loss is that they believe it isn't because they are in a trance during the process – but this is not true; some people have experienced self-hypnotizing themselves without any assistance from another person.

It has been my experience that self-hypnosis is one of the best ways to do what you want to do. Many people have reported that self-hypnosis has allowed them to overcome their fears and take the steps necessary to reach their weight loss or other health goals.

One of the advantages of using hypnosis for weight loss is that it does not require much preparation – it can be as easy as brainstorming a few suggestions or writing a few affirmations on paper – and you can use hypnosis up until you reach your goal weight.

When using hypnosis, let your imagination help guide you. I remember that the first time I used self-hypnosis, I chose to loose weight – but my idea of "lose" was very different than what most people mean when they say "lose weight." I imagined myself as a kid that was not weighed at the doctor's office – and the weight was hanging off me. That seemed to work well for me.

It is very important to keep in mind that whatever you do will have to be agreeable with your subconscious mind. This means that you need to pick suggestions and tasks which are compatible with your personal goals, personality, values, and beliefs.

If you cannot tell your subconscious mind exactly what is important to you, it will not be able to respond as well as it could otherwise.

It is also important to understand that the power of suggestion may work for or against you; if you are using self-hypnosis for weight loss, life-changing a suggestion into your subconscious mind about something that goes against, or does not fit with, your goals can cause problems.

This means that it is very important to understand that when you are using hypnosis (or any other process for personal growth), the suggestions and tasks having to do with weight loss need to fit well with your personality and lifestyle choices. A person who loves exercise will have different suggestions than a person who hates exercise. You need to be able to distinguish what is important to you and what is important to your subconscious mind.

As an example, if a person hates exercising and being in the heat, he or she will not be able to feel pleasure from being out in the heat. This would mean that the person would not have emotional reinforcement for doing it – they would simply find it unpleasant. The last thing a person wants is unpleasant feelings, so they will avoid doing it, which means that they will not get any pleasure from it. So the person's goal of weight loss goes unfulfilled by self-hypnosis because all of their suggestions do not fit with their personality and lifestyle; they have been unable to change themselves into someone who enjoys exercise.

This is one example of how a person may be able to change their thinking and feelings, but is unable to use self-hypnosis for weight loss because the suggestions do not fit.

What many people think about when they use the idea of self-hypnosis for weight loss is what happens in a dream. In a dream, you can have very realistic images and scenarios; humans do not often know that they are dreaming while in the middle of it. A person who is dreaming is able to feel emotions in a way that he or she would normally be able to while awake. When a person falls asleep, they are no longer in full control of their environment; their thoughts are no longer in full control. This is how the idea of self-hypnosis for weight loss can be used, because you are able to think about it and feel good emotions about it while dreaming, however there is one major problem with this. You may think that you are dreaming when you are in reality.

In order for a person who has never tried self-hypnosis to be able to use it for weight loss, there needs to be a way to tell the difference between true and false hypnosis. The following are things that you should be aware of that will help you determine if your hypnotherapy session is genuine or not.

At the very start of your session, the hypnotherapist should tell you exactly what hypnosis is and what a hypnotic trance really is. This will help ensure that you know how to go into a state of true hypnotic trance.

You will be asked to visualize something like a clock or an hourglass while counting backward from ten. This visualization helps relax the mind and focus on one single point, which serves as a gateway to reaching the deeper state of true hypnosis. Most sessions usually end with a final minute countdown from ten to one before your eyes are opened again.

A hypnotist can use his or her voice during a hypnosis session, but most prefer to use music or soft background music. This can help you to become very relaxed and relaxed; most people report that they don't want the instructions to sound like they are being given by a foreign language in the middle of their mind.

A hypnotist will also have his or her own methods of inducing trance; each person has different ways of going into trance. Some prefer one thing, while others prefer another. With hypnosis, if you feel that something is not working or is not what you expected, then this is a sign that your session will probably be false.

The best suggestion is to go into self-hypnosis with an open mind; it works for most people because it is able to help them learn how they think and feel about their goals. By using hypnosis, you are also able to change your subconscious mind in ways that are completely natural and beneficial for others.

When I first started doing hypnosis work, I was very alarmed by it – the idea of putting someone into a trance scared me so much that I only worked with people who were desperate for help and needed alternative methods due to being highly allergic to medicine.

Eventually, I was able to overcome my fears and do hypnosis work for people other than myself. I realized that many of the techniques used in hypnosis can be used to help heal and change other people – along with myself.

A lot of people who work with hypnosis are amazed at how quickly their lives can improve and how much they can learn by simply changing their behaviors. Many people who have never tried hypnosis realize that they have been watching television, doing things that do not fit with their beliefs and values, or simply being in a way that does not benefit anyone else as much as it could.

I think that the most important thing to remember about hypnosis for weight loss is that the suggestions you give your subconscious mind should fit with your personality and lifestyle choices. If you are looking for a way to do something that is completely out of character for you, then it will not work – even if you are in a hypnotic trance.

If you use hypnosis correctly, then it will allow your subconscious mind to make changes – allowing you to feel better about yourself and lose weight naturally. Use positive affirmations and suggestions during hypnosis, and it will help change your behavior for the better, allowing you to lose weight naturally without putting yourself through torture exercises in order to "lose weight.

If you are looking for a way to change your mindset, then hypnosis is an excellent tool. Hypnosis can be used to help you change your thoughts, feelings, and behaviors without requiring you to go through any added stress or discomfort that will hold you back from reaching your weight loss goals.

In order for self-hypnosis to work, the suggestions have to be agreeable with the subconscious mind. For weight loss purposes, this means that whatever your subconscious mind accepts as healthy is what it will eventually make a part of your lifestyle choices. In order for self-hypnosis for weight loss to work, all of the suggestions have to fit with the person's personality and lifestyle preferences.

If you are trying to change someone's lifestyle choices, then you may not be able to use hypnosis until the person wants to change their behavior. This does not mean that you cannot use self-hypnosis for weight loss, however.

It is important to understand that you cannot force your subconscious mind to do anything that it does not want to do – even if you are in a state of self-hypnosis! What this means is that if your subconscious mind is not agreeable with your suggestions, then it will not allow them to take effect. It will literally do everything in its power to reject the suggestion.

If you are using self-hypnosis for weight loss, the first thing that should be done is to create a list of suggestions and tasks which will help you reach your weight loss goal. The list should contain things that fit with your personality and lifestyle – including the things that you like to do, and the things that you do not like.

Self-Hypnosis Sessions

Self-hypnosis sessions are a great way of dealing with things like depression, anxiety, and stress. That's why they're widely used to help people lose weight.

The obesity epidemic is getting worse in many places around the world. It's not just a problem for couch potatoes - it's a scourge for those who work hard physically and subsist on healthy balanced diets as well. However, there is a solution: Hypnosis has been proven to be an effective way of losing weight fast because it eliminates the struggle someone would have if they tried to diet without hypnosis or guided meditation sessions first.

The interesting thing about hypnosis for weight loss is that it actually changes how the body handles food. By first going into a deep state of relaxation, the brain becomes receptive to any suggestions that you give it, including suggestions that your body will start burning excess fat leading to weight loss.

Here are some benefits of hypnosis:

Less craving for sweets or other junk food. You will find yourself eating healthier as well and making better food choices - such as eating more meals with lean proteins like chicken and fish, fruits, vegetables and whole grains. You will also learn to stay away from processed foods in general since they do not help with weight loss.

Increased motivation. This is a great way of boosting your drive because you will be focusing on the reasons why you want to lose weight.

More energy. Hypnosis will help increase your physical energy levels as well as make you more alert. You will also find that you don't need as much sleep, which is good considering that increased metabolism means more calories burned and less fat stored.

Losing weight can be very difficult for some people - especially those who have tried in the past to no avail or who had success but later gained all the weight back again when they returned to their old ways. There's no reason you should have to go through that.

This self-hypnosis session can be both an easy and effective tool for weight loss. It's going to focus on several different techniques, including guided meditation and deep relaxation.

It will help with a variety of health problems, including:

Post-surgical healing, such as after bariatric surgery or injury. This is just one example of the many situations where this hypnosis session will give you a significant advantage over other weight loss methods. It can also help with anxiety and depression because it puts your mind at ease by eliminating negative thoughts from it as well as helping you deal with stress due to things like work or family issues. You will discover that you have more control over your life and that things always work out.

Stress management. This is a very important part of stress - it not only causes body-related symptoms such as poor sleep, but also affects mental health, making you more prone to depression and even triggering suicidal thoughts in some people. This session can help you deal with stress better no matter what's going on in your life so you can find peace of mind again.

Whether you're currently following a weight loss plan or trying to lose weight for the first time, this hypnosis session is perfect for you. The other weight loss methods might work for you in the beginning, but they won't help you when it's time to lose the weight permanently. This session will not only help you lose weight but also keep it off so it doesn't come back again.

It is one of the best ways to stop overeating and lose weight. They are described as self-directed sessions where you enter into a state of relaxation in order to access your subconscious mind. Guided meditation is also an effective tool for weight loss because it trains the brain to be focused on thoughts about stopping eating. Gastric band hypnosis, which is a special type of hypnosis only for people that have had gastric bands, counters these negative feelings and helps them break their bad habits with food.

Self-hypnosis session had been researched in depth over the last few decades, and have proven to be an effective weight management tool for many.

More than half of the research on hypnosis has focused on weight loss. Some studies have reported a weight loss of over 45 pounds as a result. This is not just because the person doing hypnosis thinks they will lose weight, but rather that hypnosis helps people to believe in themselves and their abilities more.

Some people are recommended for gastric band hypnotherapy, where they are hypnotised into believing that their stomach is emptier than it actually is – which can reduce how much food you want to eat. Gastric band surgery is very costly and can also be difficult to reverse if you want to eat larger meals at some point in your life.

It is still a commonly held belief that hypnosis cannot be used to treat eating disorders, but there is no evidence to support this.

Hypnotherapy has been shown to be an effective treatment for those who suffer from excess eating. There are various uses of hypnosis that may help people manage their weight. Some of the more common approaches include:

Gastric banding: A non-invasive procedure where a plastic device is wrapped around the stomach and fastened to the rib cage in order to create a small pouch in which food is prevented from entering the stomach. This procedure not only helps with weight loss but can also reduce intense cravings and "hunger pangs.

Hypnosis for weight loss: Hypnosis is a safe and effective way to help people lose weight. It is important that hypnosis for weight loss be given by a trained professional, otherwise it can be hard to achieve desired results. Hypnosis for weight control should be used in conjunction with healthy eating and exercise habits.

Hypnotherapy can also help you deal with emotional issues that contribute to your overeating. If you are unsure of the reasons behind your cravings or overeating, hypnotherapy might allow you to explore some of these underlying issues that may be causing emotional distress. This can lead to a healthier relationship with food, and less emotional eating.

Hypnotherapy can help you become aware of the relationship between food and emotions, and can also help you deal with stress. If you are stressed about your impending deadlines at work, your depression after a breakup or an upcoming vacation, hypnosis for weight loss can help you find another outlet for dealing with these emotions.

You might not even know that food is a way of coping with certain situations. When you discover this, you can use other methods to deal with emotional pain and distress. Once these issues are no longer a factor in your life, it will be easier to focus on eating healthy and exercising.

When you think of self-hypnosis as a weight loss aid, you might automatically think of the stereotypical images of an overweight guy sitting in a chair with his eyes shut, completely unaware of his surroundings. Although it helps to clear your mind and focus on a relaxing state, this isn't the case with hypnosis. In fact, studies have shown that hypnosis can increase your level of awareness and help you become more focused on your goal(s).

Additionally, hypnosis is useful in helping you deal with emotional issues behind overeating such as food cravings and lack of hunger control. It can also be useful in helping you break unhealthy eating habits and motivate yourself to incorporate regular exercise into your daily routine.

If you are new to the world of weight loss, then you might not know what stage of the process is right for you. Self-hypnosis can be used in all stages, from diet selection to weight loss and maintaining a healthy weight.

So if you're looking for a proven way to help you lose weight more effectively, consider trying self-hypnosis as a weight loss aid today.

Below we've reviewed 5 different products that are all recommended as top choices when choosing self-hypnosis as a method of losing weight. We've also provided a brief introduction to guided meditation and gastric band hypnosis to help you choose the best product for your needs, which we'll look into in more detail later. Enjoy!

Find Out: Best Diet Program Of 2016 (Paleo/Keto)

How To Use: Make sure to use headphones with light music on low volume so you can focus on the sound of your own voice. It is recommended that you listen to these recordings in the evening before bed. Start by practicing deep breathing techniques as well as sitting quietly and focusing on your breathing patterns throughout the recording. Try not to think about anything else, and just listen to each track completely without looking at any notes or text other than the titles.

Meditation Benefits: If you're not sure what meditation is, then rest assured that it's one of the oldest forms of relaxation. It was practiced in Eastern cultures for centuries and has recently become a new form of treatment for anxiety and depression. Watch What I Eat Diet Plan

How To Use: You should begin by taking a few minutes to relax in a quiet place where distractions are at a minimum. Then simply listen to the recording as it guides you through an audio meditation session. The use of soothing background music will help you to relax even further and reduce stress levels.

Gastric Band Hypnosis Benefits: Gastric bands are most commonly used as a weight loss tool in European countries such as the UK. Traditional gastric bands are inserted surgically under your skin, and act as a restrictive force on the stomach.

Results Of Gastric Banding Surgery: The results of gastric band surgery are typically permanent. The band typically takes effect within a week after the procedure is finished, and can be worn for up to a year afterwards.

How To Use: It's important to start by taking it slow if you're not used to using any weight-loss tools like this one or Gastric Banding Surgery. After the first few days, you can progress from 1-2 hours per day to 3 – 4 hours per day over weeks to months.

Weight Watchers Benefits: Weight Watchers is a popular weight loss program that encourages people to exercise, make healthier food choices and be very clear on their goals.

How To Use: Weight Watchers is all about understanding what your personal goals are and helping you reach them. The program consists of weekly weigh-ins and a points system that calculates your body weight and total daily calorie intake. It's easy to use, requires no prep time and helps keep you accountable for your results.

Hypnotherapy For Weight Loss Benefits: If you're new to the world of hypnosis then it might be overwhelming to think about trying it out. However, hypnotherapy is one of the most effective ways of losing weight and controlling your cravings, and is typically used by people who already use other methods. You should start by doing any online research you can find to learn about the process and see if you like what you read before starting a program.

How To Use:For beginners, it's recommended that you download a recording on your phone or mp3 player so that you can listen to it while out doing other things. The recording should be at least 15 minutes long, as it depends on how much thought needs to be put into the session.

Results Of Hypnotherapy: The results of hypnotherapy are typically permanent. However, you should still use other weight loss methods along with it to help with motivation as well as weight maintenance.

How To Use:It's recommended that you only listen to guided meditation recordings for 1-2 hours per day. Feel free to take breaks if you feel overwhelmed or don't like the way you feel during the recording, but be sure to finish the session at least two days per week. Start by practicing deep breathing techniques and then sit quietly with your eyes closed as the meditation track guides you through pleasant imagery and relaxation training.

Benefits Of Mindfulness Meditation: Mindfulness meditation is one of the more recent forms of meditation, and is used as a way to help people with chronic pain as well as anxiety and depression. It's recommended that you practice mindfulness meditation once per day for at least 15 minutes each session, but once you become more experienced with it you can build your sessions up to 30 minutes long.

How To Use:It's not recommended that you listen to guided mindfulness meditation tracks every day. Instead, start by using it for 10-15 minute sessions daily and then build your sessions to 30 minutes over time. You should focus on breathing techniques such as deep breathing or slow abdominal breathing during the recording.

Benefits Of Guided Dreaming: There are many people who feel uncomfortable or even afraid of their dreams. Guided dreaming is a type of hypnotherapy that helps you to fully explore your dreams, accept them and gain a better understanding of them. Guided dreaming recordings should be listened to before you go to bed at night and can help you sleep more deeply than normal.

The Power of Guided Meditation

The power of guided meditation and its benefits have been documented for centuries. It's packed with an incredible number of benefits, from increasing creativity to relieving stress and aiding in sleep. Guided meditation has been scientifically proven to be at least as powerful as medication for depression and anxiety.

This book explores the power of hypnosis for weight loss, including some success stories and how it can work for anyone.

What is the hypnosis for weight loss process?

The Guided Meditation Hypnosis for Weight Loss Process, while it uses hypnosis, doesn't actually place you in a hypnotic trance. Instead, it gets your subconscious mind to focus on the positive change you want to make in your life. It will help you to achieve your goals, and have all the amazing benefits of lower weight and increased fitness.

How Guided Meditation Hypnosis Can Help You Lose Weight...

Over time, this altered state of focus will lead your subconscious mind to accept that it's OK to lose weight. You'll start to think about food in a new way, and with a new attitude towards healthy eating.

Think of your subconscious mind as a small child, completely trusting of those around it, and easily influenced. If you make sure it's in the right frame of mind, then you can give it the positive eating habits you want.

How to do guided meditation hypnosis for weight loss

The Guided Meditation Hypnosis for Weight Loss Process is incredibly easy to learn. In fact anyone can do it, whatever your fitness or weight goals may be. The process is as follows:

Set aside around 10-20 minutes a day for meditation Set up an altar or create an area which you associate with inner peace (a little like a mini-shrine). Get in a comfortable, relaxed position. Sit or lie down if you can, and don't worry about closing your eyes. Focus on your breathing, and on stilling your mind. Try to clear your mind of all thoughts and worries – just briefly focus on where the air enters and leaves your body. When you're ready, start reciting the affirmations for focused meditation in a relaxed tone of voice. these resound statements affirm what you want to achieve, helping you build belief and positivity regarding weight loss. They should be said slowly but clearly – don't worry about specific phrasing or rushing through them too fast – just read them at a normal pace. Each affirmation should be said twice, for a total of 8-12 times:

1. I am now focused on the positive change I want to make in my life...

2. ...the purpose of this is to help me reach my fitness and weight goals...

3. ...that will help me live the most healthy life possible, and stay strong and fit...

4. ...and become healthier with every passing day...

5. I can achieve all the weight loss goals I want to, effortlessly...through hypnosis for weight loss...

6. ...without any negative effects on my health or wellbeing...

7. I am now ready to begin this process...

8. ...by reciting the Guided Meditation Hypnosis for Weight Loss Process...

9. ...which will help me achieve my fitness and weight goals...

10. ...and all with the help of hypnosis...for weight loss...

It's really that simple: just follow these 10 steps, once or twice a day, and you'll be on your way to achieving your goals in no time at all.

A few Guided Meditation Hypnosis for Weight Loss Tips

While the above method is easy to do, it's also important to make sure that you're doing it properly, so that you get the most out of the hypnosis weight loss techniques. Here are some guidelines for achieving your goals.

Before you begin your meditation, take a few minutes to center yourself and calm your mind. Take some slow breaths, focus on relaxing every muscle in your body, and let go of all stress and tension.

The first step in doing this should be to find a quiet spot for yourself with no distractions. The ideal is a place which you feel comfortable, which is free of other distractions and noise.

Find an area in your home where you are comfortable. Choose one area of the room that doesn't need activity, and put a couple of cushions down if you would like to take a relaxed pose. Make this an area of relaxation for yourself, as it will allow your mind to settle into the positive space. If you have trouble choosing a spot, try looking around your house; any place could be fine to use for this process – just check to see if there are any distractions or interruptions such as loud noises or light sources.

There are different types of meditation; choose one that is most suitable to you. This process can be useful in a number of different ways, and you're not limited to doing it as a form of guided meditation hypnosis. It's simple enough to do, and it can help you focus on weight loss in the right way. You may then use Guided Meditation Hypnosis for Weight Loss Techniques whenever you need them.

Benefits: How Guided Meditation Hypnosis Can Help You Lose Weight...

The benefits of Guided Meditation Hypnosis for Weight Loss are many. They include:

Better focus and concentration – A lot of people find that using guided meditation hypnosis techniques relaxes their mind and body, allowing them to concentrate fully on the task at hand. It's easy to lose focus when carrying out weight loss exercises, but using hypnosis can help you think about what you are doing and achieve results more quickly.

– A lot of people find that using guided meditation techniques relaxes their mind and body, allowing them to concentrate fully on the task at hand. It's easy to lose focus when carrying out weight loss exercises, but using can help you think about what you are doing and achieve results more quickly. Relaxation – Guided meditation hypnosis doesn't just help with concentration; it also helps with relaxation . When you use relaxation techniques to calm your mind, it allows stress and tension to leave your body. You can then concentrate better, and support the weight loss process more easily.

– Guided meditation doesn't just help with concentration; it also helps with relaxation. When you use relaxation techniques to calm your mind, it allows stress and tension to leave your body. You can then concentrate better, and support the weight loss process more easily. Control over eating habits – If you're a person who loves food but is struggling with weight issues, then you may find that Guided Meditation Hypnosis for Weight Loss helps you to control your eating habits. As you become more aware of your body you can start to make better choices about what to eat.

– If you're a person who loves food but is struggling with weight issues, then you may find that helps you to control your eating habits. As you become more aware of your body you can start to make better choices about what to eat. Increased energy – When your mind is relaxed and focused, it's easier for energy levels to increase. This means that instead of being tired and lethargic all the time, it will be easier for you to be active and carry out exercise routines.

– When your mind is relaxed and focused, it's easier for energy levels to increase. This means that instead of being tired and lethargic all the time, it will be easier for you to be active and carry out exercise routines. Feelings of euphoria – You may find that when you are using meditation to lose weight, you feel relaxed and happy. Meditation can help with both short and long-term weight loss, but it's best to try this with a professional before making big changes in your eating habits. Guided Meditation Hypnosis for Weight Loss or Mindfulness Meditation ?

It's important to speak with someone who is trained in the art of hypnosis, especially when you're using Guided Meditation Hypnosis for Weight Loss or Mindfulness Meditation . The reason is that hypnosis can be an extremely powerful tool, and therefore, it's important to use it correctly.

That being said, you can learn a lot from a professional; they can teach you how to use hypnosis in the best possible way. They are also able to help you with answering your personal questions about Mindfulness Meditation or Guided Meditation Hypnosis for Weight Loss – all this will help you lose weight faster.

Hypnosis for Weight Loss – the Benefits

The advantages of hypnosis for weight loss are numerous. First of all, it has been proven that using hypnosis helps you focus on your goal. This means that you won't be distracted by things like hunger or cravings anymore. It's a good thing because those two things can easily influence your success.

Another advantage is that through hypnosis, you can learn how to create new habits, as well as how to kick out bad habits. You will focus on positive behaviors and learn how to develop healthy eating habits which will help you lose weight and keep it off for good.

You will also learn how to maintain a healthy lifestyle through visualization, which can help you deal with stress better and reach your goals in the long run.

Is Guided Meditation Hypnosis for Weight Loss Safe?

The answer is yes – it's 100% safe to use Guided Meditation Hypnosis for Weight Loss. This means that you don't have to worry about doing it in place of other habits or solutions. In fact, it's considered an extremely safe way of developing healthy behaviors.

People all over the world have lost weight and kept it off without any negative effects on their health or wellbeing due to this process. There have been many cases of people being able to achieve their fitness and weight goals without any negative effects on their health or wellbeing, which is why it's considered one of the most effective ways of weight loss.

Hypnosis and Weight Loss – Does It Work?

The answer is yes, hypnosis for weight loss really works. This means that you don't have to carry out any kind of exercise routine or diet plan; you can get started with hypnosis for weight loss very quickly. You'll lose weight fast because the positive mood it creates will make you feel motivated to reach your fitness and weight goals.

– Does It Work? The answer is yes, hypnosis really works. This means that you don't have to carry out any kind of exercise routine or diet plan; you can get started with hypnosis for weight loss very quickly. You'll lose weight fast because the positive mood it creates will make you feel motivated to reach your fitness and weight goals. The use of guided meditation techniques can help you control your eating habits; instead of eating mindlessly, you will learn how to slow down and focus on what food you are eating. This process will help you develop healthy habits, which are essential if you want to lose weight.

Guided meditation hypnosis for weight loss can help you relax. When you are relaxed, it will be easier for your mind to communicate with your body and influence it. This is important because when your mind and body work in tandem, you'll have a better chance of losing weight in a healthy way.

Meditation for Weight Loss – The Truth About Hypnosis

Using the power of hypnosis is no longer an issue; in fact, it's considered one of the best ways of weight loss. It's easy to learn how to do hypnosis techniques yourself, and you can do them with anyone no matter where they live in the world.

What people don't understand about hypnosis for weight loss is that it can be used for a number of different things. It can help you with developing healthy habits, as well as with improving your concentration and focus, while reducing stress and negative emotions.

It's a really good way of supporting weight loss, and it doesn't leave any room for doubt when it comes to using hypnosis to lose weight because it has a lot of benefits for the user. These techniques aren't just good for helping you lose weight – they are also designed to help you improve your health in general.

– The Truth About Hypnosis is that it can be used for a number of different things. It can help you with developing healthy habits, as well as with improving your concentration and focus, while reducing stress and negative emotions. It's a really good way of supporting weight loss, and it doesn't leave any room for doubt when it comes to using hypnosis to lose weight because it has a lot of benefits for the user. These techniques aren't just good for helping you lose weight – they are also designed to help you improve your health in general. Hypnosis is not going to work on its own; you are going to have to use some of the other techniques like Guided Meditation Hypnosis for Weight Loss or Mindfulness Meditation. If you take the time to learn how to use these techniques, you will be able to get really good results.

While the use of hypnosis alone is not going to be enough for attaining your weight loss goals, it can definitely help support and improve your lifestyle in many other ways. There are so many benefits when you combine hypnosis with other techniques; it's a good thing that you have this type of information at your disposal.

Guided Meditation Hypnosis – Weight Loss in Less Time with No Stress!

Recognizing and overcoming stress is essential for weight loss; Guided Meditation Hypnosis is a powerful tool which will allow you to relax and enjoy this process. Hypnosis is an excellent way of dealing with stress, and can help you understand how to deal with it better.

Having a negative attitude towards losing weight is one of the biggest challenges for many people who want to achieve these goals. If you're looking for a strong and effective way of dealing with your weight loss, then try Guided Meditation Hypnosis; this process will allow you to overcome stress and do it in the safest way possible.

It's done in such a way that you are able to use this technique at any time – whether you are feeling stressed before going on vacation or just before going on a date. Guided Meditation Hypnosis helps you develop positive habits which will support your weight loss goals.

Deep Sleep Meditation Techniques

Deep Sleep Meditation Techniques are a very powerful and very effective technique for getting deep relaxation, which is often needed for achieving the level of deep sleep required to lose weight. Deep Sleep Meditation Techniques are also great for any other time you need to get a deeper level of relaxation.

Consistently achieving deep sleep meditation takes practice, especially if you've never done any deep sleep meditation exercises before. In fact, most people won't be able to consistently achieve deep sleep meditation on their first day of trying. Fortunately, there are a few tips and techniques you can use to make it easier and less frustrating when practicing your deep sleep meditation exercises.

The first thing to realize is that it's normal that you might not be able to get into deep sleep every time you try. It's important to not dwell on it and keep trying, but if you give up after a few nights of trying, you'll never make it. You need to be patient about getting into deep sleep. Many people will have sessions where they aren't able to get into deep sleep, but then have other sessions where they do.

One thing that can help with making your deep sleep meditation exercises easier is using hypnosis (or meditation). Hypnosis is a way of focusing your thoughts so you can achieve a deeper level of relaxation than you would normally be able to without hypnosis. Hypnosis can help reduce your stress and your anxiety about achieving deep sleep and because of this it will make it much easier for you to achieve relaxation in general.

The next thing is something that you'll find out about very quickly during your deep sleep meditation exercises – hunger. If you're getting hungry, it's likely that you're in the middle of a deep sleep meditation session and it's not the time to be eating! You have to make sure and not eat or drink anything for at least an hour before you engage in a deep sleep meditation session.

Another thing to remember is that because of these hunger pains, if you stop mid-way through a deep sleep meditation session, sometimes it can take several minutes for your body to realize that and stop being hungry. This can make it difficult to go back into deeper levels of relaxation once you've stopped. It's a good idea to practice your deep sleep meditation exercises at least once per day. It doesn't have to be for more than 10-15 minutes, but it's something that is worth doing.

What are the Different kinds of Deep Sleep Meditation Techniques?

There are many different kinds of hypnosis and meditation exercises, but there are only really two main types: Deep sleep and Supernatural (or Self-Hypnosis). Both of these types have their advantages and disadvantages, but in the end the main factor determining which one you will prefer is your individual preference.

There are other types of deep sleep meditations, but the Deep Sleep Meditation Techniques that I will be going over are the ones that I think give you the best results. The first type of deep sleep meditation is called Prophetic Hypnosis. Prophetic hypnosis is a technique developed by Michael Phillips which translates pretty much directly into English as 'hypnotic prophecy'. It's important to realize that although you can use prophetic hypnosis to gain some amazing insights into your life as well as figure out exactly what it is you want in life, it's not a particularly effective way to lose weight in and of itself.

Prophetic hypnosis does involve some relaxation techniques and if you're using them to lose weight this can be very helpful. The reason that the hypnosis is called prophetic is because it will explain what you're about to experience in your present-day life, what's going to happen and it will predict the future for you so that you can avoid the negative events in your life and put yourself at a better position. It's important to realize that this isn't a weight loss technique and if your main goal is weight loss then using prophetic hypnosis wouldn't be such a great idea.

The second type of deep sleep meditation is known as Supernatural Hypnosis. This technique involves being asked a question (often several times) during a state of deep sleep. You then answer the question in your mind while you're in a deep level of relaxation which helps to program your unconscious mind to do what it is you desire. Supernatural hypnosis is a very effective weight loss technique. It's important to realize that although it's one of the most powerful hypnotic techniques, it can be one of the most difficult ones as well. The reason for this is that there are several elements at play during a session and sometimes these elements will conflict with each other or distract you from focusing on what you're doing.

It involves immersion or repeating a thought over and over particularly during the state of deep sleep . This allows for an easier focus and helps really get into your subconscious mind.

What are the Advantages of Deep Sleep Meditation Techniques?

The great thing about deep sleep meditation techniques is that there are many different kinds of them. There is the Prophetic Hypnosis which can help you predict your future, there is the Supernatural Hypnosis technique which can help you program your desires and most importantly there is what I call 'Path Creation' (or Pathway Creation). This technique involves using your senses to create pathways for yourself during hypnosis.

Pathway creation allows you to create a path in your mind for yourself to follow (or visualize). All it requires is that you imagine yourself going through an exercise and then put in the sensations of actually doing it.

I've seen many people take this to the extreme. They'll create a route that shows where they are going, what their car looks like, what the weather is like, and so on. This can be quite addictive for some people as you can visualize yourself doing something which will make you feel an incredible sense of achievement.

The other advantage of pathway creation is that without it you will feel lost and confused during your deep sleep meditation sessions. This is because without a pathway to follow, you will often forget what it is you are trying to achieve during these sessions. The advantage of having a clear pathway that you can follow makes the whole process far more enjoyable and fulfilling.

What are the Disadvantages of Deep Sleep Meditation Techniques?

The main disadvantage that I've come across with deep sleep meditation techniques is that too many people use them as an excuse to not work out (or do anything for themselves) in their day-to-day lives.

One of the main reasons for this is because you don't feel as though you're actually working out. There is no real sense of 'exertion' or 'effort' involved in your work out when using deep sleep meditation techniques. You simply lie down, repeat something over and over again, go to sleep and wake up to continue with it all over again the next day.

However, I strongly believe that if you know what your goals are in life and you have a clear path that you can follow then there should be no excuse for not following through with them. You should not simply use this method as an excuse to not do anything.

The other disadvantage (and this is more so for people new to the idea of hypnosis) is that you can develop a sense of apathy towards your deep sleep meditation techniques. Essentially, when you start using them you'll be excited. You'll feel like they are truly going to change your life and get you the body that you want. But after a while that sense of excitement will wear off and you will no longer believe in it all as much as you used too. If this occurs then try listening to motivational videos while using your deep sleep audio tracks.

If you have a clear path that you want to follow in life then you will be able to follow through with it. You will feel excited about it and not see a reason why you wouldn't complete your goals, because they are yours. But if you don't have a real sense of purpose in life then I don't see how deep sleep meditation techniques (or any other type of hypnosis for that matter) are going to be of any use to you.

This is the main reason why I loved using the Deep Sleep Meditation method by Dr. Wayne Barber. It gave me a sense of something to look forward too. There was something that I knew that I was going to accomplish and that made staying on track easier for me. I'm not saying that you need to buy the whole program (which is recommended) in order to find this purpose, but what I am trying to say is this: find out what your purpose is in life and follow through with it. Find out what your goals are for the future and follow through with those goals. That way you'll have a reason why you need to meditate every night and why you need to stay on track.

What is meditation?

To be honest, it's a complete "duh" question seeing as it's the main reason why people want to learn it (or have questions about it). So let me try and help you understand what meditation means.

Meditation is a form of controlled relaxation that is used to help you control your mind and body in order to achieve a deeper level of relaxation or calmness.

Have you experienced one of the following?

-Depressed Mood?

-Depression?

-Anxiety and Stress Symptoms such as: irritability, difficulty concentrating, insomnia and feeling tense or panicked.

-Excessive worry about events or activities that may not occur for months or years in the future

-Sleep problems such as insomnia and waking up during the night.   -Thoughts of suicide that have passed through your head, but you didn't act on them.

If so, then it is natural to ask how can hypnotherapy help me? It's a way to control your thoughts so they are more positive. It is also a way to control your emotions and hopefully get rid of your worry and anxiety. When you have a hypnosis session with me, I will help you realize your true potential. Sound too good to be true? I can help you make things happen in life.

If you are a patient of mine, whether on the phone or face to face, I will ask you about the above symptoms but also how I can help. You can decide which solution would work best for you when we begin our session, as well as which type of problem that you are struggling with. You may have more than one symptom and you may be able to relate to more than one solution. As an example, I had a client that was going through a divorce and he was suffering from stress anxiety. So we came up with a solution that tackled both issues, which were insomnia and stress.

It's time to stop making excuses for not achieving your goals.

You will learn lifestyle changes that will help you achieve your goals and dreams now, as well as in the future.

You will get to the bottom of why you have been struggling with these issues and traumas in your life.

You will learn to use affirmations, self-hypnosis, guided imagery, and deep sleep strategies.

You will be taught practical ways to establish a positive mindset.

You will learn how to use your subconscious mind and even the unconscious mind. You will discover how you can make your thoughts, words and actions become reality. You will discover how you can get rid of your fears and anxieties that have been holding you back in life forever. For example, I had one client who was going through a divorce but was suffering from sleep problems as well as depression symptoms such as feeling hopeless, irritable and anxious. We came up with a solution that tackled both issues as well as stress anxiety that this client was dealing with.

You can find yourself once again. Once you have achieved your goals and become the person within that you desire to be, life will open up great opportunities for you.

I am a powerful hypnotist, effective coach, and a lifestyle expert who wants to help you create the changes in your life that will bring you more success, happiness and fulfillment. As your coach I will not only guide you from where you are right now but also inspiring and motivate your future success.

Meditations for Relaxation and Self-Image

The following two scripts are intended to work together. While the first one is designed to lead you into a deep relaxation state, the second to focus on your self-image. Since the own self-image is a belief implanted in our deep subconscious, a state of deep relaxation will allow you to manipulate it more effectively. However, if you are confident with relaxation techniques and you know how to relax rapidly, you can skip the first script and jump directly to the second one.

Script 1

To get into this meditation, make sure that you are keeping your eyes closed and focused only on falling asleep. For the remainder of the meditation, we are going to use "I" statements. Remember to think of these thoughts as they come into your mind as if they were your own. As we count down from ten, make sure to focus on your breathing, and making your body as relaxed as possible.

Ten, nine, eight, seven, six, five, four, three, two, one.

I can feel my body get lighter and lighter as I relax my muscles and melt into the bed. I can tell that my body is tired and needs to be relaxed at this point. It is important that I nestle myself into bed so that I can better get the rest I need to start the day off tomorrow.

As I start to become more and more relaxed, I feel like my bed is turning into a cloud. Each breath I let out, I feel myself relaxing more and more. The air that I breathe in is energy that's going to help me feel even more relaxed.

As I breathe in, I feel all of the things that happened to me today, but as I breathe out, I let these thoughts go and pay no more attention to them. As I'm breathing in, I accept all that has happened to me today, and as I breathe out, I let go, knowing that holding onto it is only going to cause me more stress.

With every breath that I let out, I feel lighter and lighter. Each time I let the breath out, I feel like I'm sinking deeper into the clouds. I know now that I do not have to carry all of the weight with me that I have been feeling throughout the day.

I can become more and more relaxed, letting myself float and become lighter and lighter. I am drifting away from my bed now, being lifted away like a big fluffy cloud. I am not afraid of anything that I might be leaving behind. I know that it is okay to drift up and away, into the sky and looking down below me.

I am drifting from all of my responsibilities. I do not have to take care of them now. They'll be there when I get back. Right now, I only need to focus on drifting into the sky and becoming relaxed. The only thing that I need to think about is becoming more tired, feeling the fluffy cloud around me that keeps me nice and cozy.

Worrying about the things that I have to do later is not going to help me feel any better now.

I do not need to really worry about this, however. It is not a pressing issue. I might not be asleep, but at least I am resting my body.

As I look down, I see all of the people that aren't yet resting theirs. They could be in bed, but they chose to be out late. They could be drifting in the clouds, sleepy like me, but instead they are staying awake, making it harder for themselves to think and function throughout the day tomorrow.

I am taking care of my health. I am looking out for myself tomorrow. By making sure that I am focused on relaxing and falling asleep, I am ensuring that tomorrow will be an easy day for me. Tomorrow I will be relaxed, because I'm making sure that I'm tired now.

Sometimes, it is hard for me to fall asleep because I do not spend enough time winding down. It can take a little longer to get fully relaxed, and I need to remember that as I'm trying to fall asleep. It will be easier for me now to fall asleep because I am paying special attention to really winding down.

I can feel my body becoming more and more relaxed as I regulate my breathing.

As I am floating above on my fluffy cloud, I can see the wind ripple through the tree leaves. I can feel that air blow through my hair, traveling gently into my lungs. As I take a big deep breath in, I can feel how this air fills me with so much relaxation. I let the wind out slowly, and I become one with the world around me. Though not everyone is asleep, I can still feel the peace and serenity that exists all throughout this beautiful sky.

As I continue to let the air enter and exit my body, I get higher and higher. Before I know it, I can see the clouds around me, making pure gray surroundings. Some stars are still twinkling through the clouds, and I can see the black night sky behind them. As I look down, I see less and less as I become enveloped within the cloud.

Where I am now, I can no longer see the cloud that I'm actually lying on. Where my original cloud starts and stops is no longer easily identifiable. I have become one with all of the clouds at this point.

I am still floating, not worried about what's going on below me.

There is nothing around, and I feel that relaxation in every part of my body. It has never been easier than it is now to completely relax and focus only on this moment.

I can twist and move my body a bit and that will change where and how I am traveling throughout the sky. I have no plan for where I'm going, however. It doesn't really matter if I go forward, backward, left or right. The only thing I care about is feeling every last ounce of my body relax.

It is not until now, when I'm up in the clouds, that I really realize just how much tension I carry throughout my body.

Now that I am here, nowhere, nothing around me but clouds, I realize that I can feel like this all the time.

Never before have I been so tired, and now I am ultimately relaxed so I can get a full and deep night's sleep.

The more that I practice going up into the clouds like this, the easier it will be to fall asleep on a regular basis. I can do this when I'm napping, if I wake up in the middle of the night, or simply when I initially try to fall asleep.

If I want to ensure that I can fall asleep easily and stay asleep, I need to relax my entire body.

The cloud is starting to drift down now, and I understand what it means to completely let go of everything that I am feeling and allow myself to become more rested.

The cloud is passing over the streets now, and I can see that so many people are focused on getting back into bed. My cloud is moving towards my house, doing all the work so that I can remain as still and calm as possible. I do not have to worry about doing anything other than becoming entirely asleep.

My cloud gently puts me back into my bed. I can feel the warm blankets around me and the soft mattress beneath me. Everything that I experienced throughout the day is over now, and I do not have to worry about doing anything other than drifting away. Everything that stressed me out is over, and what waits tomorrow is beyond anything I can predict.

I can still feel my eyes become heavier; my breathing slower. When I reach one, I will be almost all the way asleep.

Ten, nine, eight, seven, six, five, four, three, two, one.

Script 2

Now that you are completely relaxed, I want you to take note of how you are feeling as a whole. How are you doing at this moment? How does your body feel?

Take a few moments and scan your body. There is no need to judge yourself right now. All I want you to do is notice is how your body is feeling from your head to your toes.

Scan through your body from your feet...to your ankles...all the way up your legs...and into your hips. At your own pace, scan your body through your stomach, chest, hands, shoulders, neck, head, and face.

As you focus on your body, notice how it begins to relax with no conscious effort. As you scan your body, feel as the muscles become looser and less tense on their own. All you need to do is lay quiet and remain relaxed. You feel happy that this is happening naturally. With each passing moment, your body falls more relaxed, even more, ready to fall asleep.

Now that you are feeling more relaxed, I want to talk about your body image. Many of us move through the day, uncomfortable, simply because we are not happy with ourselves and the way we look. But what is body image? Are you thinking about what your body looks like? Perhaps you are thinking about the ideas you have about your body. How are you feeling about your physical self at this moment? What does body image mean to you?

Inhale...and exhale...

As you continue to focus on your breath, I invite you to take a few moments to consider the thoughts and ideas you have about your body. How do these thoughts make you feel as you scan over your own body image? For some, you may feel comfortable and content. For others, you are unhappy, unaccepting, or dissatisfied. Perhaps, there is a combination depending on how kind you are to yourself. However, you feel, accept the emotions you are feeling at this moment.

Stay with me for a moment. I invite you to ponder how it would feel to accept your body the way it is? How would it feel to be okay with your physical self? Take a few moments now to breathe, and picture in detail how this would feel.

Breathe in...and breathe out...wonderful.

Now, try to think of a moment in your life when you accepted your physical self. Whether it be your whole self or a part of yourself that you really enjoy, think of a moment.

Which part of your body do you accept?

Imagine now, how it would feel to accept your whole body as opposed to thinking of yourself as a collection of separate parts. If you are beginning to feel stressed out over these thoughts, allow us to take a few steps back to return to relaxation.

Notice certain parts tensing up at this moment. Make a note of these locations and focus positive energy to return these body parts to total relaxation. Inhale...and exhale...you are safe and loved at this moment. You are calm and relaxed...inhale...and exhale...

When you return to a state of total relaxation and calm, I invite you to repeat the following body image affirmations after me. If you don't feel like repeating these, try to listen and relax as I speak. As you work on a positive body image, you may feel less stressed throughout the day. When we love ourselves, it grants us the ability to spread that love to others. Perhaps if you loved yourself more, you would take the time to release stress and enjoy a peaceful night's rest. Who knows, perhaps your body image has been bringing you down more than you ever imagined.

When you are ready, repeat after me. Each affirmation I am about to say is entirely true. Even if you don't believe it, you will work through your negative thoughts until you believe them to be so. Let's begin.

I am perfect the way I am.

(Pause)

I choose to accept the way I am.

(Pause)

My body is acceptable the way it is at this moment.

(Pause)

I choose to accept the body I am in.

(Pause)

I am a wonderful person as a whole.

(Pause)

There is no reason to be perfect.

(Pause)

I have imperfections, and that is okay.

(Pause)

I love the person that I am.

(Pause)

I am human, and I have flaws.

(Pause)

I choose to accept these flaws.

(Pause)

I will stop judging my body.

(Pause)

I am in love with who I am.

(Pause)

I choose to accept myself.

(Pause)

I love myself so that I can love others.

Wonderful. Feel free to repeat these affirmations as often as you need. Now that we have gone through some, how are you feeling? Whatever you are feeling at this moment is perfectly acceptable. Perhaps you believe every word I have told you, and perhaps you don't. As you practice positive body image more, you may find yourself becoming less stressed and much happier.

Inhale...and   two...and   three...and   four...and   pause...two...three...and exhale...two...three...four...five...

You are doing wonderfully. In a few moments, we will be moving onto exercises so you can fall asleep. Before we get there, I want you to turn your focus inward. Take a deep, truthful look inside to find your authentic self.

As you do this, begin to reflect on your values. What is important to you? What do you value most in life? Why is it that you chose this audio to help release stress so that you can sleep better at night? For the next few moments, I invite you to focus on your breath and ask yourself these very important questions.

(Pause)

Breathe in...breathe out...

What is left when you strip all of these problems away? This person is who you are at the core. All of your character traits and personality makes you who you are, and that is all you can ask of yourself. You work hard. You are a committed person. You are in love with your life.

With all of these positive changes you have made in just one night, it is time to put your mind to rest. You have done a wonderful job of working on your well-being. At this moment, you are feeling calm and relaxed. You have let go of your worries, explored your true self, and found your authentic core. When you are ready, take a deep breath in and let it go.

At this moment, you should feel completely calm and at peace. Your body begins to gently tell you that it is time to fall asleep. In the next few moments, we will begin to place your mind and soul at rest. You will sleep peacefully and deep through the night. In the morning, you will awaken feeling calm and well rested at the time you need to wake up.

The Power of Positive Daily Affirmations, Benefits

The first step to weight loss is often just getting started with a healthier lifestyle. The trick is doing it in a way that feels good. Don't worry - you don't have to feel bad about your past or yourself when you're doing this. It's all about setting up healthy habits that will last the rest of your life and leave you feeling good! Of course, too many people say "I know I should be eating better" or "I KNOW I need to exercise more. But somehow, they never get around to it.

How do you motivate yourself?

Try positive daily affirmations as a way to kickstart your new healthy lifestyle. There are many ways to use positive affirmations. For starters, write out a list of what you want in life. What would make you happy? Include everything from "I want more money" to "I want to find my soul mate". Think big and write big! Positive affirmations work best when they're written in the present tense as if everything is already happening! When we write in the future it can seem like we're putting it off and that somehow derails us from actually doing it.

What are some positive affirmations for weight loss?

Here are some examples of positive affirmations to use in order to get slim:
I exercise regularly. I eat what I need to stay at my ideal weight and feel great. My body looks amazing! I lose weight easily, naturally, and effortlessly. My appetite is shrinking along with my waistline! My clothes fit better than ever. I am the healthiest and happiest that I have ever been in my life. I am a radiant being of health. My body is healthy and strong. Every day I feel better than the day before. I am easy on my body, and it's easy on me too. I eat slowly and mindfully, which helps me to avoid overeating and lose weight. I eat what I want in moderation and my body doesn't complain. I have the energy to be a leader, not a follower. I enjoy my new healthy lifestyle! I wake up feeling energized and excited for the day ahead!

By creating positive daily affirmations, you're giving yourself permission to create your own reality. You can be overweight or thin and still feel great about who you are. And that doesn't mean that you have to spend all of your time thinking about your weight or trying to force yourself into a slim body.

This is a great exercise to do every day in order to keep you motivated and inspired!

What is the best way to use positive affirmations?

Positive affirmations work best when they're used daily, and at least twice a day. The more you do it, the more powerful your results will be. This can also be a great tool for motivation and inspiration, so it's easy to incorporate into your day. Just remember to be consistent and positive! You can read through your list of positive affirmations early in the morning if you want and then later as part of your long term plan throughout the day.

Here's an example of how you can use positive affirmations for weight loss:

I am easy on my body, and it's easy on me too. I eat slowly and mindfully, which helps me to avoid overeating and lose weight. I eat what I want in moderation and my body doesn't complain. I love exercising regularly. I have the energy to be a leader, not a follower. My clothes fit better than ever. I love to exercise! It is easy for me to find more time for exercise every day. I am the healthiest and happiest that I have ever been in my life.

What are the benefits of positive affirmations?

Positive affirmations work well because they can help you express your true desires. Now this doesn't mean that you need to spend all of your time thinking about your weight. In fact, a lot of times when we feel bad about our bodies we completely shut down and stop telling ourselves what we really want! By writing out your list of positive affirmations it helps you to become more creative and open with yourself, which is often the key to unlocking your true self-worth. It's also the key to changing any negative thinking into something more positive and empowering. This is a great reminder of what you want, and a great way for you to kickstart your new healthy lifestyle.

How many positive affirmations do I need to say?

It all depends on your own personal needs. Some people say one a day and that works for them. Others might say more than one every day. Try it out and see what feels good to you. Your personal experience with positive affirmations will vary, so it's best to experiment for yourself.

What is the best way to use positive affirmations?

One of the most important things about using positive affirmations is that they are completely in your control! You can use them in any way you want throughout your day or even throughout your life period.

What are some downsides of positive affirmations?

There isn't any downside to positive affirmations. They work because they're simply a way to focus your energy into something positive and imaginative while keeping other aspects of your life in balance. By focusing on things that are constructive such as exercise, eating healthy food, and making healthy choices you'll eliminate some of the stress that can come with negative thinking. As the stress goes down, so does the weight! You can also use this as a tool to help you deal with uncomfortable emotions without having to do it alone.

With the aid of these very different approaches, an individual can pinpoint their personal strengths and weaknesses and work from there to find all the benefits they're longing for. All in all, these three forms of therapy have shown us a way out of the pit of depression. Meditation is extremely popular these days, and for good reason. It's an easy and efficient way to relax that really does wonders to the mind and body alike. What makes the benefits more powerful is that it's one of the most simple methods out there, but one that people generally ignore and overlook as they seem too obvious to use. Many people will dismiss either weight loss hypnosis or guided meditation because they seem "dubious". They'll have the attitude that it's too good to actually be true. What they fail to realize is that it's not the methods of inducing a trance that is questionable. It's what's in your head when you're in a trance. Meaning, if you have a bad mindset before entering, then you're doomed to fail and feel more motivated when you leave.

Gastric band hypnosis can also help people who have had an eating disorder or who simply wish to lose weight. After all, those who suffer from obesity are already more likely to feel depressed and down on themselves than those who are average weight or underweight. When you lose weight, you'll feel much more confident in yourself because of the improvement and this will make it easier to carry through with daily affirmations.

Hypnosis is not a quick fix. It takes time, concentration, and dedication. However, if you put your heart into it, you will be successful and reap the benefits of having a new outlook on life.

A growing number of people are using this or similar methods - which include hypnosis, guided meditation and gastric band hypnosis - as a way to lose weight and improve their health.

A study published in the journal Clinical Obesity found that those who underwent gastric band hypnosis lost 5.75kg more than those who only received standard counselling on diet and exercise, as well as reporting that they consumed 2,500 fewer daily calories.

This form of therapy (and many others) seems to work because it targets the subconscious mind. It helps you stay focused on achieving your goals by focusing on positive thoughts during a session.

This way, you become more motivated and you begin to naturally think in positive ways. Here are some interesting facts on how this therapy works:

1. You eat less--According to research published in the Journal of Occupational Health Psychology, if a person eats a meal before hypnosis, they may eat up to 45 percent less than after it.

2. It's easier to eat healthy foods--When people are in a state of positive thinking during hypnosis, they have an easier time making decisions that will bring them closer to their goals.

3. It helps you resist urges to over-eat--In a study published in the journal Appetite, researchers concluded that a person who undergoes hypnosis is more likely to avoid giving into temptations.

4. You'll feel better about yourself--According to a study published in the journal Obesity Surgery, patients who underwent hypnosis felt more confident and less embarrassed when they had to undergo tests associated with their treatment program.

This research has proven that this positive state of being can lead to enhanced weight loss and improved health overall.

5. It helps you lose weight--According to a study published in the International Journal of Behavioral Nutrition and Physical Activity, those who underwent gastric band hypnosis lost 17 percent more weight than those who got standard therapy.

6. It can be used to treat depression--A study published in the journal Obesity Research examined research that looked at whether or not hypnosis could help people with depression. The results concluded that brief hypnosis sessions could make a difference for those struggling with mental illness.

7. It's an effective treatment for binge eating--Another study found that patients who were undergoing gastric band surgery could be helped by having hypnosis sessions before and after surgery. The therapy helped them to learn the reasons why they ate so frequently.

8. It can help with stress--In a study published in the International Journal of Clinical and Experimental Hypnosis, researchers found that this form of therapy can help people deal with chronic stress and anxiety.

With these benefits, it's no wonder that more and more people are turning to this method as a way to lose weight and have a healthier lifestyle.

9. It can help you gain confidence--Studies have found that those who undergo gastric band surgery are more confident in their new physical appearance. They also experience a feeling of being more attractive and more in control of their life.

10. You won't get bored with it--The results from the study published in Obesity Research indicate a positive trend for people who undergo hypnosis while on gastric band surgery, as they're able to better handle the stresses and anxieties associated with losing weight.

11. It's safer than surgery--Some people think that gastric sleeve or banding surgery is unsafe because it can lead to potential complications such as bleeding and infection, which could cause death if not treated properly.

Research has proven that this form of therapy is much safer, as it does not require a surgeon and therefore can be done by a physician of any kind. Even though the results are not as drastic, they're still effective.

12. It's less invasive--According to the journal Obesity Research , gastric band surgery is a much more invasive procedure than hypnosis, so the therapy seems to be safer for those who undergo it.

13. You'll experience faster weight loss--Another study published in the International Journal of Clinical and Experimental Hypnosis concluded that patients who underwent gastric band surgery lost almost twice as much weight as those who didn't have hypnosis sessions at all during or after their surgery.

14. It's simple to do--Hypnosis is a very simple and easy form of therapy that can be done right at home without any effort.

15. It's a great option for individuals who have health issues--It's important to note that anyone can benefit from this type of therapy, regardless of their health issues.

In addition, the energy used during hypnosis sessions is less than what would be needed during surgery or counseling programs, so it helps save precious energy in order to get the results you want faster than you would if you had surgery or went through regular therapy.

16. It's less expensive--People who undergo hypnosis sessions are often happy to know that it can actually save them money.

With the cost of surgery being so high, many people are turning to hypnosis as a less expensive option for weight loss.

17. You won't have to miss work--Hypnosis allows for more flexibility with your schedule while giving you the same benefits that gastric band surgery offers.

18. You'll be more confident and feel better about yourself--According to research published in the Journal of Psychosomatic Research, people who underwent hypnosis felt more confident about having surgery and had better control over their eating habits after they completed their sessions.

19. It will help with your sleeping--If you're tired or stressed right now and are unable to sleep, hypnosis can calm down your mind and help you get the rest you need.

20. It will decrease anxiety--Research shows that people who undergo hypnosis for weight loss have lower levels of anxiety than those who didn't go through it at all.

List of Positive Daily affirmations for Weight Loss

List of Positive Daily affirmations for Weight Loss

Are you struggling with your weight, or going through a midlife crisis? You don't have to worry any more. There are many tools for weight loss available in the market now and they work wonders!

The latest and greatest weight-loss technique is using hypnosis for getting rid of stubborn fat areas in a jiffy. This can help you boost metabolism as well as recover from healthy eating habits which may be difficult to follow on your own. In addition, it will enable you to indulge in all those sugary and fatty foods that have been banned from your diet without feeling guilty about it.

So how can you achieve a weight loss success, without feeling like your entire life is spinning out of control? These hypnosis audio weight loss scripts are your solution. You will actually feel like you are having a conversation with a friend, while relaxing to the soothing tones. Even if one of these audios isn't exactly what you're looking for we have plenty more that deal with overcoming depression, releasing stress and anxiety, improving self esteem and preventing alcohol abuse.

Using hypnosis for weight loss has become extremely popular over the past few years. It's now known that when you use meditation to set an intention, whether that be losing weight, quitting smoking or quitting drinking, your subconscious is able to work on fulfilling your wishes without any effort on your part.

Following are some of the positive affirmations for weight loss:

I look in the mirror and I like what I see. I am smart enough to understand the importance of managing my diet. I make time for exercise every day because it makes me feel good. I am starting a new way of eating today and in two weeks, my body will thank me.

I am a confident and happy person who knows that I deserve to be successful in all aspects of my life. I deserve the best in everything that I do, whether it is my health, social life or work. I appreciate my body and give myself the time, attention and nourishment it needs to feel its best. I look forward with joy, excitement and anticipation to a world where all people are truly seen as equal regardless of size.

I am guided by love for myself as well as for others on their own weight journey.

My self-care includes practicing healthy eating habits that support me living an active lifestyle which includes daily exercise at least 30 minutes per day 5 days per week (including these structured workouts). I do this because I believe that I will feel happier and healthier!

I am diferent from other people who struggle with their weight, because I choose to live a healthy lifestyle.

By embracing my goals and by enjoying everything that life has to offer, I feel more relaxed and in control. My body is beautiful, healthy and vibrant.

I feel delicious! I love all of the foods that I am eating and the way that they make me feel.

I am a person of excellence. I deserve to be treated well and to treat myself well.

I learn my lesson quickly, every time!

I don't care what others think about me! My body is my temple and I will not let anyone or anything keep me from living a healthy life.

My health is my priority, so it is important for me to eat healthy foods that are low in calories and fat and high in nutrients.

I can maintain an exercise program that is healthy and sustainable in my life. My nutrition is balanced, my waistline is trim, I feel energized, and I am happy!

My body is no longer a weakness, but it is a source of freedom and joy.

My body, mind and spirit are connected in an indivisible whole. All three aspects of myself are 100% healthy and powerful together!

Dieting will only make me feel worse once I reach my goal weight. I can maintain a healthy lifestyle that supports my weight loss goals.

I am strong and powerful with my physical, emotional, and spiritual health.

My body is an amazing and miraculous machine that can heal itself.

I deserve all the nourishment that this beautiful world has to offer me!

I'm going through tough times right now, but I know that with faith, patience, and perseverance all things work together for good in my life.

I am grateful and happy! I begin my day with gratitude for the bits and pieces that make up my body. I appreciate how my body can perform every single day without failure. My body is a miracle machine, and I am honored to be able to witness its wondrous capabilities.

Everyone has a right to be healthy, happy, vibrant and at peace with their bodies.

My mind, soul and spirit are healthy and vibrant.

I love my life! My body is beautiful! It's the work of God! He designed me this way for a reason. I thank him daily for creating me out of love.

I love myself! I accept myself as I am.

Today's a new day! I will begin my day with a positive attitude.

The journey to weight loss is not easy so it's important for me to focus on the present moment. I put my mind in a happy place, focus on what is ahead of me, and try my best to enjoy the journey!

Today is the first day of the rest of my life. I am standing up for myself and taking control over my life and body.

My thoughts will change once I lose this weight, but until then, all that matters is how beautiful and powerful I am right now, in this moment.

I am strong and beautiful just the way I am!

I now have the health, vitality, and mental strength to do what it takes to achieve my weight loss goals.

I am fulfilled by practicing a healthy lifestyle of nourishing myself in all ways: physically, emotionally, and spiritually.

To build a world where everyone is seen as equal regardless of size.

I deserve to be loved and respected for who I am rather than for what I look like.

I accept myself as being worthy of love and belonging in this world.

I am now willing to experience everything life has to offer.

I am in love with myself! I have come so far and I cannot wait to see what the future holds for me.

I am open-minded, intelligent and have a wisdom that is outside of this world.

All of my stress and worries are melting away as I reach my weight loss goals.

All of the joy in my life flows through me, dropping pounds effortlessly all day long.

I have the courage to change my eating habits today and choose a healthy lifestyle.

I am a spiritual being living in this physical world. My body is a sacred temple that needs to be respected and nourished.

I am grateful for all of the lessons I've learned from my past experiences with food and fitness.

My health is my priority, so it is important for me to eat healthy foods that are low in calories and fat and high in nutrients.

I have the ability to maintain an exercise program that is healthy and sustainable in my life.

Every thing we own has some emotional attachment to it

.A new outlook does not take time

.A new outlook will improve every aspect of your life

.Affirmations are a powerful tool to change your perspective and transform your life for the better

.Collective conscious help you helps us, as well as others, so long as you make it a habit to think good thoughts about them

.If we want something bad enough, we can always make it happen with the power of positive thinking and affirmations for success on our side

.Have a positive attitude and you are sure to succeed

.Have a great day!!

Every thing we own has some emotional attachment to it.

A new outlook does not take time.

"A new outlook will improve every aspect of your life."

"Affirmations are a powerful tool to change your perspective and transform your life for the better."

Collective conscious help you helps us, as well as others, so long as you make it a habit to think good thoughts about them.

If we want something bad enough, we can always make it happen with the power of positive thinking and affirmations for success on our side.

"Have a positive attitude and you are sure to succeed."

Have a great day!!

List of Positive Daily Affirmations for Weight Loss and Worthiness (for every major area of your life)

Like Star Light, I shine bright!

I am an A-grade student who makes my parents proud.

I am a super Mom /Dad.

Like, Sun light I shine Brighter to help the world be great.

I live in a clean environment to sustain my good health.

I love myself and accept myself just the way I am... Nobody else has that power to determine how well or how bad I do in any given situation.

I always fulfill my needs and desires through responsible and disciplined use of money.

I overcome fear of my own insecurity and the judgments of others because I know that I am a worthy human being.

I understand that people will always care about me so long as I keep on living authentically.

I use this powerful tool to help others when they feel helpless.

I am responsible for my own life and control my body independent of outside influences.

"I am confident in myself, and the choices I make are based on authentic values. As long as I remain calm and focused, everything else will work out fine.

This post features positive daily affirmations for weight loss. Affirmations are a powerful tool that you can use to change your mind and make healthier choices. You can also use them to overcome any limitations you may have put on yourself like "I am not worthy of success." Affirmations are an effective way to stay motivated and keep moving forward when things get tough. Use these affirmations and make them your own as you work towards lasting weight loss goals.

1. In the next hour, I will be more mindful about what I eat which means I will enjoy my food better, feel better afterwards, and have a smaller waistline as the result!

2. I have the power to change my waistline! I don't need anyone else to help me reach my goals.

3. I will not be a victim of my taste buds or food cravings! I can choose foods that help me feel stronger, lighter, and healthier.

4. If a certain food isn't helping me meet my weight loss goals, then I won't eat it again!

5. When I eat foods that support my weight loss goals, it feels so good! It feels like a special treat that tastes delicious and makes me feel good about myself.

6. I will not stop my efforts to succeed at weight loss until I'm down to the number I've wanted for a long time.

7. During this weight loss program, I will be able to say no to tempting foods that may cause me to binge!

8. I can find strategies that make eating healthy and living a healthy lifestyle easier for me!

9. No one can stop me from achieving my goals! The only person holding me back is me!

10. My attitude could always be better so allow it the chance to improve instead of trying to push through as if nothing is wrong even when things are not perfect. Holding on too tight could cause some problems in the long run.

11. I deserve to look and feel my best.

12. I have the power to change my life for the better!

13. It doesn't matter who does or doesn't believe in me, all that matters is that I believe in myself!

14. When I'm with other people, I will not use food as a way of connecting with them!

15. Every day, as soon as possible, I will update my weight loss journal so that I can stay focused on what's important and never forget what's working for me and what isn't!

You deserve the best

Your weight is perfect for you

You are strong and capable

The tools that you need will show up for you when you need them most, even if it seems like they won't. You just have to stay committed to your changes and keep moving forward.

You are worthy of good health, happiness, and love.

Visualization: How to do it?

In order to achieve a goal, it is vital that you visualize yourself succeeding. Remembering past achievements can also help you succeed in the future. This book will teach you how visualization forces your subconscious to do what it thinks is necessary for success.

You can practice visualization to achieve goals in different parts of your life. Say you want to set new, weight-reducing goals and shed some extra pounds. One of the first things you must do is visualize yourself achieving this goal; imagine the look of satisfaction on your face as you achieve your target weight. If you are trying to recall where an item might be, visualize where it is and remember exactly where it is located.

The Key: Setting a goal and visualizing yourself achieving that goal will help make that goal more attainable; your subconscious mind will know what steps need to be taken for success.

How to Achieve Your Goal: Visualize your goal and follow the steps that will make you achieve it.

Visualize how you will feel after achieving your goal - it can be better than you ever imagined. After seeing yourself achieving your goal and feeling satisfied, visualize what will need to happen for success. Say that you want to lose 10 pounds in 2 weeks, but have a difficult time doing so; your subconscious mind knows that the most efficient way to reduce body weight is through diet. So visualize losing 10 pounds of body weight in 2 weeks, along with how you'll feel afterwards- euphoric, confident and happy! The more realistic you make these visions, the closer they'll come to becoming reality.

Replace negative self-talk with positive self-talk:

Most people allow their subconscious mind to control them. If you tell your subconscious mind that you're fat and cannot achieve a goal, it will start believing these lies. But if you tell your subconscious mind that you're going to succeed, and picture yourself achieving what you want, your subconscious mind will know the steps needed for success.

Here's how it works:

You're walking from your car into a shopping mall and you see a pair of jeans that are too small. You automatically start to say, "Oh, I'm so fat! I'll never be able to fit into those pants!" But then you stop yourself and remind yourself that you will soon fit into those pants. You visualize yourself in that pair of jeans and imagine the satisfaction on your face as you zip up your favorite pair of pants.

Your subconscious mind will remember this positive self-talk and will strive to make it a reality. If you practice positive self-talk, replacing negative comments with positive ones, it won't be long until the negativity stops and the positivity begins.

It all starts with a vision of what we envision for ourselves - and then the process of making it happen. You want to be healthier, more attractive, or maybe just more motivated! Whatever it is you want to change about yourself, you first need to clear your mind from any negative thoughts and create an active imagination that will motivate you to take action.

Hypnotherapy is both a science and an art form which looks at the subconscious mind in order to find solutions for problems such as overeating, compulsive behavior including sex addiction or other addictive behavior with drugs, smoking addiction or alcoholism.

It is the best way to lose weight with hypnosis because it is a permanent method and you will be able to keep that weight off for good. Hypnosis helps you not only lose weight but also gives you great benefits.

With hypnosis, you will be able to control your appetite, which means less cravings for food and sweets. Hypnosis helps you understand your body better by understanding the connection between emotions and behavior. By using hypnotherapy, it allows you to find out why you eat certain foods during certain situations. With this, it allows your brain to let go of the cravings so that you can have more control of yourself and stop eating over emotional situations.

Actually lose weight with a hypnosis diet

Hypnosis works much better than a hypnotherapy because it is easier to follow through with the hypnosis method. You have to have your own mind made up in order for it to work and not give up. If you want to lose weight for good you will need to keep yourself motivated and think positive thoughts throughout the day. If you want to stop smoking, then you need an active imagination by thinking of how your life will be better without smoking. Remember, positive thoughts are what sets us apart from others and that is what makes a difference in our lives.

How to do it?

The first thing you will need to do is prepare yourself. You will want to have a quiet and peaceful place where you will not be disturbed at all. When people are bothered by sounds, phone calls or anything else, it can take away your concentration, which means that hypnosis won't work as efficiently. You also want to be comfortable and not too hot or too cold. Hypnosis is done in a relaxed state where you are the most comfortable. Also, if you have a headache or feel sick for some reason then it may affect your session negatively as well. Don't assume that hypnosis is an instant cure for cancer or something like that because not everything works for everyone the same way.

Have all your materials ready before you begin. You will need a chair for you to sit on, a quiet place where you can sit comfortably and have no distractions, and some specific things that will trigger the memories from your subconscious.

You are going to want something that is an object or a person that reminds you of something negative or upsetting from your past, such as someone who hurt or betrayed you (a parent, teacher, lover or friend). You are also going to want to visualize yourself eating the food that is causing the problem with compulsive behavior. Also have something in mind that makes it more likely for these objects or situations to show up again in order for you to recognize them during hypnotherapy.

How to start?

Begin by sitting down in a comfortable chair and close your eyes. Breathe in slowly and out just as slow. You will want to inhale through your nose and exhale through your mouth. You need to stay relaxed so that you don't wake up from this hypnosis. If you feel like you are about to fall asleep, then open your eyes for a moment and continue breathing deeply. After a few minutes of this, you should be relaxed enough to continue with the original breathing exercise.

You will want to talk about whatever you have in mind for the session and let your imagination go as far as it wants. Any memory that you think might be related to your weight loss goals will help the hypnosis work more efficiently for you.

Now, you will want to think about the things that are causing problems with an extreme weight loss hypnosis. For example, if you are trying to lose weight because of issues from childhood, then you would want to visualize something from those times that is causing this problem. If someone is still bothering you, then visualize yourself fulfilling your desires by satisfying your every need.

You can keep on doing this until you feel like it is working but be careful because you don't want to fall asleep. If you feel like you are about to drift off into sleep, then open your eyes and return to the original breathing technique for a few minutes.

Then, close your eyes again and visualize the people or situations that are bothering you in any way (related to weight). You will want to describe what they look like as if you were watching them through a camera lens. Imagine yourself as a bigger and more powerful person than everyone else around you so that nobody can bother you or make fun of you for anything. This will help you keep a positive outlook on everything and help you to lose more weight.

You can do this exercise as long as you are comfortable in order to get the most out of your session. To finish your hypnosis off, you will want to return to the breathing exercise and then focus on what the people or situations look like around you. Concentrate on what they are saying and take note of how they look around you. They might be smiling but inside they are hating themselves because they know that they can't do anything that might upset or anger you. You want to feel good about yourself so visualize them standing there with nothing but happiness for yourself.

After you are done, you will want to open your eyes. Stay in this position for a minute and then slowly move yourself out of the chair. Walk away from it and leave your session, gradually coming back to the point where you started this process. If you are comfortable, you can take a few moments to write down anything that is stuck in your mind so that later on when something comes up that triggers it, you have a way of remembering why and how these things occurred. You can do this later after your session is over or anytime during the day when you feel like it.

Remember that the most important part of any weight loss hypnosis session is following up with your own exercise and healthy eating habits. You might feel like you have to get back on track right after the session, but this is not really true. The best way to help yourself is to get started as soon as possible. That way you are more likely to continue feeling good for a longer period of time rather than going straight into temptation and temptation related issues.

Just keep in mind that there are no quick fixes for your weight loss goals and you need to take it easy with yourself if you have slipped up. Listen to your body and make sure you are not pushing yourself too hard at times. If you need to take a break from regular exercising, that is perfectly fine. Trust me, you will be so grateful for every day that you have taken off and then when it comes back around, you will be pushing harder than ever!

Lastly, remember that weight loss hypnosis is all about making small changes as opposed to nothing. You are not going to lose a huge amount of weight without having put in the effort beforehand. These are simply suggestions and tactics for your own benefit so that they become second nature. You can use these principles on their own or in combination with other programs like an exercise routine. Either way, they will help and make all the difference in your life. You might also want to check out weight loss hypnosis and fad diets.

If you have been struggling with your weight, it is time to make a change! Weight loss hypnosis can be the push that you need to finally get started on your own weight loss journey. If this sounds like something that you would be interested in, then just look around here for some great ideas and strategies for getting rid of that extra weight once and for all. After all, the sooner you start, the sooner you will be seeing results.

Self-Esteem Exercises

Many people who are overweight or obese have low self-esteem. The reasons for this can range from a negative self-image to anger, guilt and shame. These feelings can make it difficult to lose weight because you might feel that you are not worth the trouble, or you might be angry with other people for taking care of themselves but being critical of your efforts to do the same thing. These feelings can keep you consuming more food than you need in order to feel better about yourself. Thus, a common question is: 'How do I lose weight and increase my self-esteem at the same time?'

Self-esteem exercises include taking care of your body, focusing on the positive things about yourself, learning to accept compliments with grace and humility, and changing your thoughts about yourself in a healthy manner. In order to boost your self-esteem and make it easier for you to lose weight, learn how to strengthen your inner voice by learning how to control negative thoughts. This process will help you forgive yourself for past mistakes and mistakes you have already made. You can also learn how to change the way that your body regulates emotions.

Begin by writing a list of your past mistakes. One by one, go through each mistake and try to recall the following: What were the circumstances of the mistake? What feelings came up while you were making this mistake? Were you angry with yourself, guilty or ashamed of yourself? Did you make more than one mistake?

Next, touch upon how these feelings affected your healthy eating habits. How did you feel about yourself afterwards? Did this feeling prevent you from enjoying healthy foods or exercising regularly? Were there any other situations where you used food to self-medicate or heal negative emotions.

Now that you have identified the mistakes that you have made in the past, examine how they have affected your diet. The next step is to forgive yourself for these mistakes. Remind yourself that God forgives you when you ask for forgiveness. He will forgive you if you let Him into your life. Be willing to let go of the past and learn from it at the same time. Forgive yourself for not being able to eat healthy and exercise regularly while making these mistakes, but learn how to do so now as a way of learning from your experiences and moving forward with your life.

Building up your Self Worth

Changing your beliefs about yourself is essential if you are to lose weight and build up self worth at the same time. You can do this by continuing with an exercise to begin to build up your self-worth. You can begin by going through each of your past mistakes and writing a list of the positive things about yourself. Try to find the positive aspects of the way that you are now, and as well as enumerate the good attributes that you still have but not yet recognized or acknowledged using compliments. Write down at least ten points that are positive about yourself, usually these should be things like intelligence, patience or independence.

You can also look at the mistakes that you made in the past and begin to assess how these mistakes that you have overcome have contributed to a healthy diet. By doing this, you will be able to see how your past struggles with weight loss are actually your greatest accomplishments. You can also give yourself praise for the things that you did well by changing your mindset. For example, instead of telling yourself that you ate too much last night, next time try telling yourself "I gained muscle while I was eating."

You can also begin to learn to accept compliments gracefully and humbly by learning how to receive compliments. For example, you could learn how to tell a joke and make a positive comment even if it doesn't sound very funny. A final way that you can increase your self-worth is by being happy when you are doing well and healthy by eating healthy and exercising regularly. You can do this by learning how to be happy when you are losing weight and taking your vitamins or supplements.

When you begin to work on learning how to change your beliefs about yourself, it is essential that you don't do this in a superficial manner or without first doing your best. It will help if you focus on one thing at a time, like learning how to build up self-worth on a specific level. If you are around other people who are also trying to lose weight, they can help you by validating the positive things about you that you might not have been able to see before. This process will help you learn how to love yourself and to value yourself.

Forgiving Others

Another way that you can build up your self esteem is by forgiving others who have hurt you or let you down in the past. Forgive those who have been kind of mean to you, or those who don't take your weight loss efforts seriously. By forgiving these people, it will be easier for your inner self to forgive yourself for mistakes that you might have made. You can do this by writing a letter to each person that has hurt or wronged you, asking them to forgive you as well.

You can also learn to forgive yourself. For example, if you realize that you have been holding on to anger against another person, you can decide to forgive them and let go of that anger. You can also learn how to let go of negative feelings and thoughts about healthy foods or exercise routines by gradually changing your beliefs about these things. You can do this by repeating affirmations during the day that tell yourself that it is okay to eat healthy snacks or obtain vitamins from natural sources. One positive way in which you can start forgiving others is by asking them forgiveness for misdeeds that you have committed against them, whether they are done intentionally or unintentionally. For example, you can forgive your neighbor by asking them to forgive you for dealing with their garbage twice instead of once when they were kind enough to provide your with a trash bin. Forgiveness is an essential part of making any change in life, and it will help you to feel better about yourself.

Getting Someone Else Involved in Your Weight Loss

The most important thing that you can do to build up self-worth is by getting someone else involved in the process of changing your beliefs about yourself. Another motivation that comes from knowing that someone else is watching your weight loss progress will be extremely helpful. Just as you will be motivated by knowing that someone is watching your weight loss, the person who is watching your progress will be motivated by knowing that they are helping you. You can learn how to get more involved in other people's lives by working on things that involve them, like volunteering at a local soup kitchen or improving relationships with neighbors and coworkers.

When you learn to accept other people's help, this can motivate you to do things in a positive manner. Instead of choosing to stay on the couch and watch television all day when there are plenty of non-toxic options available, you can use your time wisely in an effort to reduce your stress levels while learning how to build up self-worth. Only by accepting other people's help are you able to build up self-worth.

Getting an Involved Partner in Exercise and Weight Loss

For some people, the most difficult thing about changing their weight is getting a partner who supports this change. It can be very frustrating when you want to loose weight but have difficulty finding someone who will help you with this goal. To get an involved partner, you need to ask someone who will be supportive of your goals and think that they know all the right answers. By doing this, you can learn how to build up your self-worth by allowing someone else to be involved in the process of making changes that will give you a healthier body.

Asking Your Parents and Other Relatives for Help

If you are having trouble getting a partner or someone to help you lose weight, consider asking your parents. Most people have the best intentions of helping their children, especially when they believe that their child is not doing well. Since it can be difficult to change your behavior because of your insecurities, ask your parents and other close relatives if they would be willing to help you build up self-worth by getting involved in some way. You can show them just how beneficial losing weight will be by letting them see how much better you feel once the pain associated with being overweight has dissipated.

The main advantage of asking your parents for help is that they are normally more concerned about you than they are with themselves. The tough part is getting them to agree to help you, which might involve a bit of convincing, but once they realize how much better you will feel once you start losing weight, they should be more willing to work with you. It's difficult asking your parents for help because at some point in time most people have had experiences in which their parents have been controlling or even abusive. However, if the relationship between the parent and child is good then this should not be a problem whatsoever. And if the parent is not able to be in control of the child or if the child wants to be on their own and assert their own personality then there should not really be any problem. I think that some people have unrealistic expectations of what a relationship between parent and child should be like and they are also afraid to just let it go and give up control

Sometimes parents can get very possessive over their children. They want to have them all to themselves. They may believe that everyone else has an equal right to spend time with them. They may feel that they are wasting their time if they spend time with anyone else (even their kids) except their spouse. They may believe that there is no point in having children unless they want to have an heir to pass on the family name and wealth. I think this is just a product of the times when it was acceptable for parents to be very possessive over their children. Times have changed and there are many other acceptable ways to raise a family. But I think that in order for this to happen, most families need to be more willing to accept change, be open minded and just let go of some of their outdated beliefs.

Many people may argue that you should be able to spend time with your family without feeling like you owe them something in return. I guess that this is true if you don't feel like you owe them anything. If a child has learned how to spend time with their parents without expecting anything in return then they will not feel the need to ask their parents for assistance when it comes time for them to lose weight.

What is Gastric Band Hypnosis

Gastric Band Hypnosis is a form of hypnosis therapy that is used to help treat obesity. In this type of therapy, the patient sits down and relaxes as they listen to soothing music. As the person falls asleep, they may also notice that their stomach feels tight or bloated while listening to comforting music. They are then encouraged to enter into a deep state of relaxation where they drift off into sleep and awaken refreshed with a new sense of self-awareness about their weight problem and how it affects their health.

What is Guided Meditation?

Guided meditation is designed for people who find it difficult to sit in silence and focus on just one thing for an extended period of time. People who struggle with attention and focus are often helped by guided meditation. This form of meditation is intentionally crafted so that it helps a patient become more focused on his or her breathing, body, mind or thoughts which brings the mind in touch with something external.

What are the different types of hypnosis?

There are many different types of hypnosis, each with their own special properties and uses. You can also combine two or more types of hypnotism to provide even stronger effects for your patients.

The following is a brief list of the different types of hypnosis:

Anchor Hypnosis – This type of hypnosis involves using imagery and symbolism to help a patient focus on certain triggers to relax. Anchor hypnosis is sometimes combined with other forms of therapy in order to help patients get even better results.

Asleep Hypnosis – This type of hypnosis involves reaching a state of consciousness that is between the present and sleep but closer to sleep. The person may still be conscious enough to respond to commands without fully entering into sleep or becoming overly relaxed.

Brief Hypnosis – This type of hypnosis is designed to help the patient enter a state of hypnosis quickly. This is useful for people who are in a hurry or just want to get some results.

Deep Hypnosis – Deep hypnosis is a state where the patient experiences complete relaxation while still being completely aware of their surroundings and their body. The person may respond to suggestions but may not remember if they fell into this state at all after they awaken.

Emergency Hypnosis – This type of hypnosis allows the patient to enter into a deep level of relaxation almost instantly in case an emergency arises that requires them to be able to react quickly. This type of technique may be useful for people who work at a high risk for injury or may be injured on the job.

Elliptical Hypnosis – This type of hypnosis is designed to help patients experience deep relaxation and deep levels of healing by use of imagery and symbolism. The patient enters into a state where they become aware that they are receiving healing while they visualize their body changing to reflect this ideal healing process. The imagery is often used to represent the person's life or as a symbol for something meaningful and important to them.

Focused Hypnosis – This is often used in team sports. It allows a player to focus on certain aspects of the game while cutting out distracting elements that might occur during the game. A common use of focused hypnosis is for a sports player to visualize themselves performing techniques and skills while blocking out the audience or any other distractions that might occur.

Group Hypnosis – This type of hypnosis involves a therapist leading a group through some form of guided meditation in order to help the group achieve certain goals. An example of this would be a therapy group that meets to work on weight loss issues by using hypnosis as part of their therapy sessions.

Instant Hypnosis – This type of hypnosis is designed to allow patients who are at risk for becoming overly relaxed or who experience panic attacks, anxiety or other similar conditions the ability to enter into hypnosis quickly while still retaining control over their body and mind.

Light Hypnosis – This type of hypnosis allows a patient to experience deep relaxation while still retaining awareness of their surroundings and their body. This form of hypnosis is sometimes referred to as "light hypnosis" or "twilight."

Long Distance Hypnosis – This type of hypnotherapy is designed to allow therapists in one location to conduct sessions with clients who are located in other locations. This process is usually accomplished by using some form of technology such as Skype, Facetime, webcam or other similar messaging communication software.

Milton Model Hypnosis – This type of hypnosis involves teaching a person about the different levels that they can achieve during a hypnotic state. It teaches the person about the different triggers, cues and positive affirmations that will help them to achieve the results that they are looking for.

Mute – This type of hypnosis is similar to anchoring hypnosis in that it involves using symbolism and imagery to help a patient focus on certain things that will trigger a state of relaxation and deep concentration. However, this type of therapy focuses more on creating emotions such as love, joy or trust rather than trying to create feelings of relaxation.

Neutral Hypnosis – This type of hypnotherapy allows a therapist or doctor to provide care for patients in ways that don't involve suggestions. It allows the physician to access a patient's deepest levels of consciousness and retrieve information about the patient's medical history. It also allows physicians access to information about specific psychological or emotional issues that may be occurring.

Ni – This is a type of hypnosis that was developed by Eneko Knudsen form the Basque region of Spain. Ni works by giving people suggestions to help them learn how to reprogram their subconscious mind.

NLP – This stands for Neuro-Linguistic Programming and it is used by some therapists and hypnotherapists in order to help patients change their mindset so they can have the results that they are looking for with regard to their emotional, physical or mental well-being.

Ongoing Hypnosis – This type of hypnotism involves the use of a therapist or health care professional who will work with a patient on any given day, week, month or year. This type of therapy often requires ongoing sessions to continue helping patients take the necessary steps to improve their overall well-being.

Passive/Active Hypnotism – The difference between passive and active hypnosis is that in passive hypnosis, the patient is unable to make decisions during a session while in active hypnosis, the patient can make their own decisions. It may be helpful for people who are considering trying hypnotherapy to know that they can always choose to allow themselves to be fully hypnotized or not depending upon their own personal preferences.

Pencil and Paper – This is a type of hypnotherapy that involves writing down positive affirmations on a piece of paper. It is generally used to help people focus on their goals and objectives so that they can take the necessary steps to achieve them.

Milton Model Phobia Treatment – This type of hypnosis therapy involves teaching people about the process in which phobias are created in order for them to realize that they can overcome fears, anxiety and other similar conditions by using this new understanding. The person will then learn how to replace their negative emotions with positive ones naturally.

Positive Self-Image Hypnosis – This type of hypnotherapy benefit people who are struggling to have their own personal identity and sense of self-worth. It is also effective for people who are having a hard time realizing their full potential in life.

Post Traumatic Stress Disorder (PTSD) – This type of hypnotherapy is commonly used by military, law enforcement, and emergency personnel who have experienced trauma related injuries or deaths in the line of duty. It is a way that they can learn how to calm their minds and bodies down so that they can feel relaxed and calm while being proactive if there should be the need come up for them to do so. Find out more about this type of therapy.

Undoing the Conditioning – This type of hypnosis therapy is useful for people who are not aware of the fact that they have been conditioned to react in certain ways. These are often seen as subtle patterns that have already formed in a person's life, upbringing or past experience. Once these patterns are worked out, people can be able to break out of this and learn how to act in healthier and more fulfilling ways. Conscious Hypnotherapy can be used to help with many different health conditions, but it is usually most helpful for those suffering from phobias, anxiety disorders, PTSD or other behavioral related issues.

Hypnotherapy for Anxiety and Phobias

Phobias are characterized by a strong fear of something, which can be something in the environment (such as a snake) or in other people. Following hypnotherapy for anxiety and phobias, a person is able to confront their fears and work through them. This opens up new avenues of learning, which helps to transform a person's life.
Once work has been completed on overcoming phobias, those suffering from anxiety disorders have many more options available to them. This means that they, too, can experience a more fulfilling and unified life!

Hypnotherapy for Addictive Behaviors

It is possible to use hypnotherapy for addiction. Addictions of all sorts are characterized by an unhealthy emotional or psychological reliance on something. This can be anything from alcohol and drugs to food and extreme sports. Once addictions have been addressed with hypnotherapy, it is possible to confront these behaviors in clear-minded ways that are effective.

Hypnotherapy for Depression and Anxiety

Anxiety disorders often contribute to depression. Labeling this condition as "depression" can be misleading, however. In this situation, hypnotherapy for depression and anxiety is an excellent choice! Hypnotherapy works on the root of the issue, which is one's state of mind. This means that a person can shift away from negative feelings, such as loneliness or sadness, toward positive emotions like hope and optimism.

Loss of a loved one is often directly linked with depression. A loss such as this can leave a person feeling incomplete and out of sorts with the world around them. Hypnotherapy for depression is often effective at addressing these feelings in an empowering and healing way.

Hypnotherapy for Weight Loss

It is possible to manipulate your weight using hypnosis! In this way, hypnotherapy helps to provide you with a positive and empowering sense of self. When you feel good about yourself and your body, it becomes easier to maintain a healthy lifestyle. This will help you stay fit and healthy, which is the best way to go!

Hypnotherapy for Past Life Regression Therapy

Past life regression therapy involves going into the subconscious mind where past experiences are stored away by the brain. This is an incredibly powerful and entirely effective way to work through past issues that have left you feeling down and unfulfilled.

The therapist will work through your issues in a gentle and safe way, allowing you to discover feelings that have been buried for many years. Do not expect to go back in time to relive traumatic events such as abuse or painful surgeries. Instead, the therapist will guide you through feelings of grief, regret or other emotions related to past events.

Hypnotherapy for Relationship Problems

Many couples struggle with communication problems. This problem can usually be traced back to childhood development of personality traits which may include being overly sensitive or negative about personal relationships. Using hypnotherapy for relationship problems, these traits can be worked on in a positive and empowering way. This will leave you with more options than to be stuck in the past and needlessly hurting your partner!

Hypnotherapy for Post Traumatic Stress Disorder Therapy

Many soldiers returning from war must deal with post traumatic stress disorder. More often than not, coping mechanisms and feelings of anxiety serve as a barrier to overcome. However, this is never impossible, as long as the person has the right support system in place.

All About Gastric Band Hypnosis

-What is gastric band hypnosis?

-Why do people seek it out?

-Are there any side effects or risks from it?

-How much does it cost?

If you've been struggling to get a handle on your weight, then you're not alone. Statistics have shown that over half of American adults are either obese or overweight, and even more alarming is the fact that there is also an astounding increase in childhood obesity among children aged 6 to 11 years old. The struggle with food can be as complex as dealing with an addiction and overcoming your fear of food. Hypnotherapy has proven effective in treating alcohol dependency, smoking cravings, drug addictions and other addictive behaviors. Now it can also help you lose weight, and maybe even prevent it in the first place.

Gastric band hypnosis is one of the most recent trends in weight loss techniques. It helps you to master your food cravings and your relationship with food, ultimately enabling you to lose weight in a healthy way. Gastric band hypnosis uses a combination of proven hypnotherapeutic approaches that will help you develop long lasting and healthy habits around food. The concept behind gastric band hypnosis is that our relationship with food goes far beyond just eating; for some people, their relationship with food becomes an obsession.

The Gastric Band is a medical device that is placed around the upper portion of the stomach and can be used to restrict food intake by controlling the amount of food that people can eat at any given time. The Gastric Band is placed on a patient's stomach via an outpatient procedure and stays in place for at least two years.

In most cases, gastric band surgery does not require a lot of weight loss before surgery is performed. Surgery is simple and patients generally recover at home sleeping in their own bed without any complications; there are very few long term complications from gastric band surgery. Most surgeries are performed through laparoscopic techniques with very little discomfort involved.

Fast food, soda and other treats can cause a large amount of empty calories. In many cases, it's just as easy to eat a delicious meal as it is to eat a greasy hamburger or cheeseburger with French fries or onion rings. One area where thin people tend to struggle is in their relationship with food. The urge to overeat is great for some people and they may feel that they are unable to control this urge.

The Gastric Band aids in weight loss because it restricts the amount of food that people consume at one time and promotes healthy eating habits. The gastric band makes it easier for patients to eat smaller meals so that they can make healthier food choices and be more conscious about their eating patterns.

Gastric Band surgery is a fairly new medical procedure for weight loss. Weight loss surgery has become very popular and many patients are now choosing the gastric band as a safe and simple way to lose weight. Gastric band surgery is one of the most affordable weight loss procedures available today with minimal risks, low risks and high success rates. The procedure can cost anywhere from $6,000-$8,000 with most insurance companies paying at least 70% of that cost in many cases.

The surgeries results are immediate and are not temporary; the actual results of this procedure will remain permanent after the surgical period has concluded. There is no need to go on any dangerous crash diets or exercise routines post-surgery. People can eat whatever they desire, whenever they desire and with the gastric band, people are able to learn how to control their eating patterns.

Results may be felt in a relatively short period of time, often within 3 months after surgery. The results of gastric band surgery vary from patient to patient based on individualized needs and goals. Many people see substantial weight loss within the first six months and some people see significant results even sooner than that.

The Gastric Band has been used successfully by many patients for many years but the use of the Gastric Band is still fairly new in our medical community. It is generally safe and effective for achieving weight loss so long as the proper diet and exercise are taken. Since it is a fairly new item, the gastric band surgery can be done in a more natural setting than larger surgeries such as Lap Band surgery.

Certain types of scarring or inflammation may cause problems with the Gastric Band. There are some minor risks to the procedure but these risks are very low compared to weight loss surgery which carries with it many additional complications like heart attack or stroke and often takes longer to recover from after major surgeries such as lap band.

Gastric Band Hypnosis is an exciting new way to achieve permanent weight loss and improve health. Despite the diet industry, not a single one of these programs is scientifically proven to work. However, they may work for some people who have trouble controlling their eating habits. We at Gastric Band Hypnosis will help you find out which programs are most effective for you.

After attending a few sessions with an experienced Gastric Band hypnotist, patients often begin to lose weight quickly. Not only that, patients also report a significant change in their attitude towards food and eating as well as dramatic improvements in their overall satisfaction with life after they have undergone gastric band surgery. Normal gastric band hypnosis sessions last about an hour, and are designed to be relaxing, pleasurable and deep. Our approach is fully customized for each individual client's needs.

Hypnotherapy combines all possible benefits of both Eastern and Western therapeutic methods in one easy system. As such it is a natural choice for people who want comprehensive care that takes into account every aspect of their mental well-being - health, coping skills, emotional stability - while still respecting their individuality with a specific focus on the issues which they have expressed the most concern or pain in their life.

Hypnotherapy is a powerful tool that can be used to help you achieve your goals. Hypnotherapy sessions work by accessing your subconscious mind. Your subconscious mind is the part of your mind that controls all of your habits.

You can use hypnosis as a tool to help you eat healthier, think more positively and make healthy lifestyle changes. Hypnosis is also helpful for losing weight because it helps you stop thinking about what you're eating as much, making it easier to ignore cravings and desires to eat unhealthy foods.

Hypnotherapy for weight loss treatment requires a highly skilled professional who has the ability to both formulate a customized plan for each client, and provide the tools necessary for success. This is why we recommend seeking out a professional who has been certified by the National Board of Hypnosis.

Our hypnotherapists have helped people to quit smoking, lose weight, reduce stress, lose sleep anxiety, manage their conditions and much more. With over 35 years of combined experience in education and clinical hypnotherapy, our team of master's level clinicians are ready to help you become the best version of you.

Welcome to our blog on hypnosis for weight loss with a focus on gastric band hypnosis, guided meditation, and extreme weight loss hypnosis. We know that there are many different opinions out there, but we want to share with you what is working for us today. So, without further ado here are the three best ways to lose weight through the power of suggestion.

First up is gastric band hypnosis in which we send you deep into a relaxed state where we encourage you to visualize your stomach shrinking down and getting rid of all the excess fat that's been making it expand in size over time.

That's really where the power of hypnosis comes into its own because we can help you to literally reprogram your subconscious into seeing a slimmer, more energized you. It's this ability that makes gastric band hypnosis so effective and why people all over the world have been using it to shed those extra pounds with such ease.

As well as gastric band hypnosis, we also offer guided meditation for weight loss and extreme weight loss hypnosis in our first three tips on how to lose weight with an emphasis on the holotropic breathwork.

Our most popular gastric band hypnosis session, the Platinum Package, has helped hundreds of individuals to lose weight. We have two packages to choose from and we're happy to offer a free weight loss hypnosis download with every session. Take a look at how easy it is to use these powerful tools for weight loss right from your home or in the office.

Gastric band hypnosis is a highly effective method of losing weight because it uses the power of suggestion on an unconscious level to direct the body into knowing what it needs in order to shed fat deposits and tone up lean muscle tissue at the same time. Gastric band hypnosis is a powerful tool that can be used to help you achieve your goals. Hypnotherapy is therefore ideally suited for people who are looking for a professional who will help them make better lifestyle choices and get results in the shortest time possible. Everyone experiences change in response to hypnosis, and in this way it differs from other forms of treatment which tend to be more one-off interventions.

We also offer a free weight loss hypnosis download with every session so that the patient can learn how they can use hypnosis as a positive tool on their journey towards weight loss and overall well-being.

The simple act of choosing to listen and follow our suggestions will help make you lose weight quickly. Our highly trained hypnotherapists can help you to identify your unhealthy habits and focus on a healthier lifestyle through the power of suggestion.

Our hypnotherapy weight loss program is all about helping you make a gradual change in your daily life and focusing on achievable goals that will allow you to achieve your desired results. We'll be there throughout your journey towards lasting weight loss by helping you to understand how hypnosis can help improve certain aspects of your life, such as how you think or feel about food, and what it is that triggers cravings.

We have two packages from which to choose - the Platinum Package and the Gold Package.

Based in London our hypnotherapy weight loss treatment is available at our Central London and West London clinics. We also offer a free consultation for all new clients who would like to find out more about how we can help you. Our team of highly trained professionals will guide you through each step of your journey to better health and overall well-being. Let us be your guide today on how to lose weight with hypnosis, now available in both Central London and West London.

Weight loss through hypnosis is one of the easiest ways to change your lifestyle and get results fast without feeling hungry or deprived like you would if you were dieting alone. We can help you to make better lifestyle choices and adopt new healthy habits through this holistic approach to weight loss.

Hypnotherapy weight loss sessions are designed to help you make better lifestyle choices which can help you achieve those long-term goals of which you are dreaming. We'll guide you on the path to weight loss with a focus on your food and eating habits and the underlying issues in your mind that influence how you think about food.

If you're currently trying every diet that's available, it may seem as if there is no viable solution. Hypnosis can give you a new perspective on what's already going on in your life. More often than not, our unconscious motivation drives our behaviour, but we can control it with the help of hypnosis.

Gastric Band Hypnosis Scripts

Gastric band hypnosis scripts are a way to achieve desired weight loss goals without the discomfort and side effects of surgery. These scripts can replace a need for surgery and can help with weight loss by helping the patient develop a healthy mindset around food and diet.

If you have tried numerous diets without success, gastric band hypnosis scripts may be the solution you have been looking for. These hypnosis scripts are used to help patients who are ill for an extended period of time to lose weight and keep the weight off. This can include people with gastric bands, patients with cancer after surgery, or those who are trying to lose weight after a major illness.

This process will usually take a few months, but it will be well worth the effort. A positive mindset toward food and diet is the key to achieving your weight loss goals. Gastric band hypnosis scripts work on a deeply rooted psychological level. Because these scripts specifically target such a complex issue as weight gain or loss, they require more than one session. They also need to be repeated until the language is fully accepted by the body.

Many people have tried gastric bands and other weight loss methods without success. Studies have shown that the hypnosis scripts encourage subconscious acceptance of these systems and give patients a sense of emotional security that allows them to go through with the process.

These scripts are used in conjunction with diet plans, exercise, and medical supervision in order to achieve results for patients who are ill or overweight. Health professionals should always consult a physician before using this type of therapy.

These scripts are also a good way to keep the weight off because they help patients develop healthy eating habits and a positive mindset toward food.

These hypnosis scripts are also beneficial for those who have gastric bands. Many people who have gastric bands do not lose weight because they overeat. Over time, their stomachs stretch and fill up with food so that it is impossible to eat enough to lose weight. Although many of these patients can still eat, their stomach will fill up quickly, which is why they gain more than two pounds a week after surgery. These hypnosis scripts are designed to help these patients control the amount that they eat and become more in touch with their hunger levels. They will then be able to lose weight by eating, no matter how much food they want.

These scripts are also helpful for patients who have major illnesses. Gastric band hypnosis scripts help these patients overcome their illness and realize that it is time to start eating healthier. Many of these patients can no longer eat healthy foods or go out and eat at restaurants because they are too weak to do so. Hypnosis can also serve as a supplement to these patients' medicine. It is important that all of the facts about the illness are explained to them before starting this type of therapy.

Gastric band hypnosis scripts are used in conjunction with other weight loss programs for patients who do not have gastric bands. Those who are suffering from obesity may also benefit from these scripts since they help the person realize that there is a problem and help them to develop a positive mindset toward food.

Some of these scripts work better than others for different people, so weight loss coaches should always consider the individual before prescribing any type of therapy. Patients who have been unsuccessfully trying to lose weight may be more likely to accept these scripts than those whose issues involve their health, such as cancer patients seeking help with diet. Sometimes this type of therapy is not for everyone. This is why it is important to test the waters before beginning a long course of treatment.

These scripts work on the deepest level possible, changing how patients view their entire existence. It takes more than just positive affirmations to get patients to change their mindset toward food and diet. This is why these scripts should be used in conjunction with other therapies, such as exercise and diet plans.

Doctors should always consult with a physician before prescribing gastric band hypnosis scripts for any type of patient or situation. The Western medical community has not fully embraced this type of therapy, so a local physician may be the best option for you.

Gastric band hypnosis scripts have been proven to be enormously successful and are a valuable part of any weight loss program. They should always be considered before going off of them. Many other factors can interfere with the effectiveness of these scripts, including poor motivation and lack of follow-through. Also remember that these scripts have been used successfully with patients suffering from severe illness such as cancer or AIDS. Using these scripts without proper knowledge can result in adverse affects on your body, so it is always important to consult a professional first. Perhaps the reason why gastric bands and other weight loss methods fail is that patients are never given a chance to accept their problem. These scripts allow them to take that first step, and from there, it is up to them to see the results of their hard work.

The best way for a patient who has gastric band hypnosis scripts is to follow all of their instructions and stick with it. If these patients follow these directions, they will see positive results within a few months. It will take time for the body to change its mindset about food, so patients should be prepared for this process before starting treatment. Also, patients must never stop taking these scripts without consulting their physician. This could have serious consequences for the patient's health.

However, these scripts are not a good option for patients who want immediate results. Gastric band hypnosis scripts work differently on each person and have to be adjusted in order to be effective. People who have a negative mindset may need more time with this type of therapy before it becomes effective. It is best to start with a short course of treatment such as two or three sessions per week and then slowly up the frequency depending on progress and how positive the patient feels about the program.

Gastric band hypnosis scripts can be used for a number of different reasons. Weight loss coaches should always consider the factors that will make the treatment work for the individual patient. It is important for weight loss coaches to give these scripts a chance, since they contain some of the most effective therapeutic techniques in today's weight loss industry.

Melanie is a writer, educator and mother with two children who likes to spend her free time writing and learning things about health and nutrition. She works with her family's winery in Sonoma County, California. Melanie blogs at greenbohemia dot com about healthy lifestyle products and parenting tips.

A gastric band is a surgically placed band that creates a small pouch in the stomach, which can cause dramatic changes in the way the body uses food. This procedure requires a doctor's prescription and must be performed by a highly trained physician under general anesthesia. They have been shown to be safe and effective when compared with dieting methods, but they are not approved for long-term use.

Loops are also known as gastric bands or the restrictive dieting devices. A loop is basically a stretched piece of rubber that is inserted on the upper part of the stomach through small incisions in the abdomen and then passed under the skin and around the stomach to create an additional pouch.

The procedure is done in a hospital under general anesthesia, but it does not require an incision through the skin. The doctor will pass a small metal wire loop around the stomach and then pull in and out to create two loops. The device is placed on the upper part of the abdomen under the skin for quick weight loss results.

When looping is used for obesity treatment, it takes several months to complete but some patients see results in weeks or even days. Looping works by creating a smaller stomach pouch, which makes it easier for food to pass through and also makes you feel full sooner.

The stomach pouch becomes the main part of the stomach and is stretched out in order to reduce the size of it through gradual stretching. The looping device is used to take up space in your stomach and it can help you control eating by feeling fuller faster.

The procedure may be painful, depending on the individual, but it is much safer than other methods of weight loss surgery. The device hangs down below the top rib and its position prevents other organs from being trapped between the device and body tissue. Also, there are fewer risks involved because this procedure does not make incisions on or near any organ.

However, there are some cases where patients complain about persistent pain and discomfort after having a gastric band procedure. In order to know how to avoid this, it is important to consult the best weight loss surgeons in Austin TX.

One way to prevent pain and discomfort after gastric band surgery is by eating food that will not lead to irritation of the abdomen. It is also important not to lift heavy objects or do physical work after this procedure because it can cause bruising of the stomach wall.

It is also important to replace your laparoscopic port if it becomes damaged or infected. You can prevent gastric band complications by using proper hygiene, taking prescribed drugs, eating the right foods and exercising regularly. The reason why there are so many gastric band complications is because of the length of operation and the fact that it is a permanent procedure. It is also important to consider that this surgery still does not correct the underlying problem with obesity.

People who have undergone this type of surgery often feel depressed, hopeless or discouraged after having their band removed. Some people have resorted to other methods of weight loss such as exercise and dieting or even extreme measures like liposuction in order to regain some sense of body satisfaction.

However, more research is being done to improve the new laparoscopic band procedures so that they provide a more comfortable way for patients to lose weight and avoid excess calories during digestion.

A laparoscopic clamp is also known as the tie band or the surgical belt. It is a staple for surgeons, but it is important to understand that it is not a gastric band. The surgeon uses a sharp hook attached to a long chain which is passed through two small incisions in the abdomen and placed around the stomach. This procedure also requires general anesthesia and incisions in the abdomen.

The device can be left in place for 2-5 years after surgery, depending on how well it works and how well the patient follows their diet instructions. However, because this type of surgery does not involve making incisions on or near any part of an organ, there are fewer risks involved compared with gastric band surgery.

Mistakes to Avoid During the Diet

Mistakes to avoid during the dieting process are costly and can include weight loss plateaus, a decrease in the body's metabolism, and even an increase in water retention. Extreme Weight Loss Hypnosis, Guided Meditation, and Gastric Band Hypnosis are three of the best ways to make sure you don't make dieting mistakes.

We'll start with hypnosis. This technique is designed to help you change the way that your brain interprets everything related to food intake. It's especially useful for those looking for a permanent change in their eating habits. The next technique is guided meditation; it teaches you mindfulness techniques that focus on saying yes only when appropriate. Mindfulness is a way of being present and focused on the here and now. Finally, there is gastric band hypnosis. This technique helps you lose weight safely because it helps you gain control over appetite. But before you can fully benefit from this hypnosis, you'll need to have a band placed on your stomach. A gastric band is designed to help people lose weight by restricting their consumption of food. So even if you don't use the guided meditation or mindfulness techniques in this guide, it's still an optimal choice for those seeking a lifestyle change that will lead them to permanent weight loss in a healthy way. Whatever your weight loss goals are, it's important that you look into each of the above techniques so that you can make sure you don't make any mistakes during the dieting process. And if you're looking to transform your body and get the results you've always wanted, then you need to make sure that you use these three techniques as a part of your weight loss journey.

This includes not eating enough calories, eating too few fats, or just not working out enough. These mistakes can lead to extreme weight loss.

The only way out of this is by using hypnosis or guided meditation to tackle the problem head on. In fact, gastric band hypnosis is one of the most effective ways to lose weight quickly and easily without all the hard work and deprivation most people have to go through when trying to lose weight.

What is the Gastric Band Hypnosis Diet?

The gastric band hypnosis diet is a unique way of losing weight that combines hypnosis and guided meditation with something called gastric band hypnosis.

The first thing you need to understand about this type of hypnosis is what it means by the term "band." The term "band" refers to a theoretical device, which in this case is a small ring, similar to an elastic band that would be placed around your stomach. This ring would then create a new barrier for ingested food and would keep you from eating as much food as you normally would.

You might be asking yourself how or why this ring got its name. Well, the official name for this device is the "Gastric Band System." The band is typically made of medical grade silicone and would be placed around your upper stomach, where it would create a barrier of sorts that keeps food from getting past your stomach.

The band is also designed to create a feeling of fullness in order to keep you from eating too many calories throughout the day.

How Does Hypnosis Fit in with this Weight Loss Diet?

The second thing you need to understand about gastric band hypnosis is that it's usually combined with guided meditation and hypnosis.

The guided meditation is mostly used for calming the mind and putting your mind to ease so that you can better reach a trance state.

The hypnosis is used to put you into a deep trance, which is where most people feel a sense of relaxation and calmness. It also helps to ensure that the gastric band system will work properly in order for the weight loss process to proceed.

What are Some Advantages of This Weight Loss Diet?

There are several advantages to using this type of hypnosis and guided meditation diet.

The first advantage is that this type of diet is very effective. This diet has been known to work very well for those who have gone through it several times and have been able to reach their goals.

The second advantage is that the diet is designed for those who want an easy way to lose weight, which works out well for the vast majority of people.

Another advantage that many people will find with this diet is that there are many different types of mind altering techniques used in conjunction with the guide who will help you during your guided meditation sessions.

Based on all the research and experience taught by professionals in the field, this weight loss diet is a successful one.

How is this Weight Loss Diet Different from Other Diets?

There are different types of diets that work for the long term and other types of diets that work for short term goals. There are also different ways to lose weight, such as the strict dieting method, or the gradual dieting method, or the gastric band diet.

This kind of hypnosis and guided meditation is unique because it allows you to find a way to lose weight where you don't have to rely on all the exercise and deprivation. The only real changes you have to go through is by simply going through guided meditation sessions while wearing a gastric band system.

And this weight loss diet is simple, easy, and quick. All you have to do to lose the weight you want is go through a guided meditation session while wearing your gastric band system.

This is a great way to lose weight quickly and easily for many people who want to lose some weight but don't want all the work and effort that comes with it.

How Soon Will I Receive Results from This Weight Loss Diet?

The speed of results will depend on how much time you put into the process by going through guided meditation sessions, which should be done at least 2-3 times per day. The more sessions you go through, the faster you will see results.

And, it doesn't matter if you're taking this diet before or after your gastric band surgery; as long as you enter a trance state during the guided meditation sessions while wearing your band system, then the slow and gradual process of fat dedication will start.

How Long Does It Take to Start to See Results?

Anyone who has used this type of hypnosis for weight loss can tell you that once you do start to see results, it's really dramatic. And for many people who have lost a lot of weight in a relatively short amount of time that is very exciting.

However, the best way to find out how fast your weight is going to start dropping is by going through a guided meditation session along with your band system. This will guarantee the fastest results.

Then following your guided meditation sessions you can simply track how quickly your body is going to lose the weight that you want to lose.

How Long Does it Take for Me to Start Dropping Weight?

The amount of time it takes for you to see results will depend on a few different factors, including how much time you invest in the program and the type of diet that you are on prior to using hypnosis or guided meditation.

People who are not overweight and are in fairly good shape can usually see results within a few days of beginning the hypnosis sessions. But, those who are severely overweight will probably have to wait a little longer. This will usually depend on how well your body is going to respond to the hypnosis sessions and how well your mind is going to be able to focus on what's being said during the meditation sessions.

The more you can clear your mind while listening to the guided meditation, the faster you're going to start dropping weight.

Avoiding Junkfoods

Avoiding junk food, exercising more, and eating less sounds like a simple solution to shedding a few pounds. But the reality of doing these things can be so daunting that many people give up before they even get started.

These three sets of recordings work in unison to help you stay on track with your weight loss goals. Whether it's hypnosis for appetite control or guided meditation intended to enhance relaxation so you're more motivated to exercise—these are all proven ways of boosting your motivation and self-discipline! They have helped thousands lose weight more easily than ever before. Eating healthy is one of the most effective ways to lose weight. But even with our best intentions, some days are better than others and we still find ourselves giving into temptation. After all, a cookie tastes so good! But what does it feel like when the sugar high wears off? You're probably not as hungry as before, but now you feel tired and sluggish. The next day, you might even feel guilty for eating that cookie in the first place. This can lead to an endless cycle of guilt and more eating. Consistently eating junk food isn't just bad for your waistline; it's bad for your health. But what if I told you there was an easy way to eat healthier?

The first thing that stands in the way of most people's goals is the amount of willpower required to make changes in their daily routine, particularly when they feel unmotivated or stressed out. For some, it's easier to skip a workout than stick with a healthy diet. But if you're already going to the gym regularly, why not make it even easier by investing in this set? It's all about setting yourself up for success. Before even starting your first meal or exercise routine, slip on the first recording and let relaxation wash over you. You'll notice that your body feels heavy and sleepy—a natural side effect of the hypnosis session. When you wake, you'll feel more energized and prepared to handle the challenges of a healthy diet and exercise routine. You will be able to think more clearly, process information more effectively, and make better decisions.

The second recording is designed to help you appreciate how great it feels when your body is in shape. It will raise your energy levels so that exercising feels easier and more motivating than ever before! You'll feel totally rejuvenated after every workout. And third, for all those who have trouble controlling their appetite, this set might just be the solution you're looking for (oh yes it is).

If you want to break through that weight loss plateau and get back on track, then you might want to look into gastric band hypnosis - an effective way to make peace with your food while still being able to eat normally.

Avoiding junk food , restricting calories, and exercising might seem like the answer. And while it can be a little tricky, these strategies are typically enough to go from overweight to healthier and fit.

However, if you have tried these tactics and they're not working for you, it's time to call in the big guns: extreme weight loss hypnosis.

Extreme weight loss hypnosis is about getting to the root of the problem and finding a more permanent solution. It's not just about dieting. That's why extreme weight loss hypnosis includes guided meditation, and hypnotherapy to turn your thoughts into actions.

In extreme weight loss hypnosis, you'll learn how eating disorders are caused by an inner need to control your body. That includes learning to accept your body no matter what. You'll also learn to relax and feel more peaceful with food.

This is a lot more than a weight loss hypnosis tape. It's behavioral modification therapy for overeating.

Guided meditation is also included in this set. It will teach you to let go of stress the moment it arises, which will help lead you down the path to better health and happiness. It's time to stop putting yourself down for the way your body looks and start respecting it for all it does! This is what extreme weight loss hypnosis can do for you.

"I was spending so much wasted mental energy putting myself down and feeling guilty about eating that I hardly had any energy left over to do anything else but eat, eat, eat — not just emotionally but physically too. I was feeling so much stress that I filled the air with tension and anxiety. It was a vicious cycle.

Avoiding junk food is difficult for many people. With so much advertising and temptation, you can often find yourself eating more than you should or even grabbing something that's advertised. That's why this post is here. It'll tell you all about the power of hypnosis and how it can help you lose weight and get healthy in a way that is easy, truly effective, and fun. It includes information on when to use hypnosis, how it works, what to expect with these recordings, and more.

There's no stopping the junk food industry and their fantastical solutions to problems that don't exist — but there are some other ways to stop eating so much! You'll be surprised what will happen if you give hypnosis a try - just listen to one of these recordings for 15 minutes or so every day! Hopefully then Junk Food Won't Taste So Good anymore.

How Much Weight Can You Lose?

The New York Times did a study on this and other similar issues. In the article, they found that a lot of people use hypnosis as part of their weight loss program. Hypnosis is a natural method to help you lose weight, it's as natural as any other way of losing weight.

It is a surefire way of helping you lose weight, but it can also be difficult. It can also be hard to get the right mindset to put yourself on a diet and workout regime. That's where hypnotherapy comes in!

We provide guided meditation for extreme weight loss, as well as hypnosis and gastric band hypnosis, all in one place. Whatever your goal is - whether it's just to tone up or to shed excess pounds - we've got you covered.

Clinical hypnosis can help you get into a state of mind where you'll be able to take things at your own pace, no matter how busy or stressed out you are all the time. If you're an athlete who's always tired and needs extra motivation to get up and go along with your training, then hypnosis can be a great tool for helping you obtain that extra edge.

There are various methods we use in order to achieve success with hypnotherapy and guided meditation. If you want something specific to achieve, we can tailor a program that will produce results for you - if this is what you're after then we should certainly talk.

If you're someone who wants to lose weight, we can put you on an audio program that will help you get into a state of mind where you'll be able to stick to the diet and exercise regime that we'll set for you.

The process is simple - first, we will have a discussion about what sort of weight loss goals you have. We'll talk about your background - your lifestyle, eating habits, activities that might contribute to your weight loss problem. We'll also talk about your current diet, and the amount of food you eat. Then we'll set out a program. You'll listen to the recording every day for a certain amount of time, and then we'll check your progress. At the end of the session, you will know whether or not you've been successful in reaching your weight loss goals.

We can also use hypnotherapy to help with affirmations and concepts that have been helping us achieve our goals already. We may use cognitive therapy techniques when we need to change negative thinking patterns to bring about positive change in the way we think about ourselves.

The Most Effective Foods to Eat to Help you Lose Weight

The most effective foods to eat to help you lose weight are green leafy vegetables, whey protein, whole-wheat bread, skim milk and natural peanut butter. The most effective weight loss supplements are Garcinia Cambogia extract, green tea extract, CLA (conjugated linoleic acid), and Alpha Lipoic Acid.

In more than half of all Americans, obesity is the result of a hormonal disorder called leptin resistance. This condition causes reduced energy expenditure and reduced satiety, resulting in an uncontrollable appetite. The most effective overweight treatments are hypnosis and other behavioral therapies, including biofeedback training and diet modification. Surgery is the most effective treatment for morbid obesity – bariatric surgery can triple weight loss rates by eliminating food intake and helping patients feel full more easily.

Low-carbohydrate diets are the best way to lose weight at any age. The Atkins diet and the South Beach Diet, known for their high protein diets, are low-carbohydrate diets that have been shown to be effective for weight loss.

Eating a small amount of carbohydrate at mealtimes is the best way to lose weight and maintain your weight loss. There's no need to count calories, or track carbohydrates. Everyone over-estimates how much they eat by a factor of about two – so if you follow a hypnosis session plan and follow it by eating less than the most extreme dieters, chances are you'll automatically stick to the "fewer calories per day" goal without even realizing it. And that means your weight will naturally start decreasing.

The most effective drug to help you lose weight is leptin. In patients with metabolic syndrome, leptin resistance plays a role in the development of insulin resistance, heart disease and diabetes. And leptin is the only drug that has been shown clinically to be able to reverse this syndrome. Leptin levels can quickly go up and down depending on diet and exercise, but it's not a major concern since it's also a normal part of our bodies physiology.

Most people have no idea that their brain literally controls their body weight, calorie consumption and fat loss – even more than any other factor. The two most important factors for controlling your body weight are: (1) your brain; and (2) how you think about food.

Sugar and starch are the real enemy of weight loss, so if you try to cut these out of your diet, your body will create its own fat storage devices so they can be stored in another location. The best way to lose weight is to reduce your carbohydrate consumption – this is the only way to lose weight without dieting or crash dieting. This is the most effective way of losing weight quickly and safely – it's more effective than any other method that has ever been created and tested by thousands of scientists worldwide.

Eliminating refined carbohydrates from your diet is one of the most crucial aspects of losing weight. This means no sugar, no bread, no corn or wheat products and very few carbs. Any kind of starch is a refined carbohydrate.

Eating more protein is the best way for everyone – from overweight people to skinny people alike – to improve their health and increase their energy levels. Protein is the most effective way to suppress appetite, help you feel full longer, burn off more calories and lose more weight while eating fewer calories. It also helps you look younger, feel stronger and perform better physically – overall it's the single most important thing you can do for your health overall.

The most effective diet in the world is intermittent fasting or 'time restricted feeding'. This is the only diet that has been proven scientifically to be more effective than any other diet. It's specifically designed to help overweight people lose weight by reducing their calorie intake by about 25% – this is done without restrictions on the types of foods they eat.

The most effective supplements for weight loss are the ones that reduce cravings and have mechanisms similar to leptin in your body. This means CLA, green tea extract, Garcinia Cambogia, ALA (Alpha Lipoic Acid) and hoodia – all of which can help reduce appetite cravings and increase energy levels.

Once you've lost fat, your muscles burn more calories than they did before you started losing fat. Muscle burns far more calories than fat – this is why you can't lose fat if you don't have any muscle. If you don't train, your body quickly loses muscle mass as well, so the more muscles you have the better.

Metabolic syndrome is a hormonal and cellular disorder that causes insulin resistance, leptin resistance, abdominal obesity, high triglycerides, high blood pressure – all of which lead to heart disease. The only effective treatment for metabolic syndrome are hypnosis and other behavioral therapies.

The best hypnosis weight loss sessions are going to be the ones that help you lose weight and change your eating habits in a way that's permanent. You can listen to the same session every day if you want – this works for most people – but the reason it works is because of how the subconscious mind works. The more consistent you are with your session plans, the easier it will be to stick with them on a long-term basis. The most effective way to lose weight is to combine all of the best methods into a single plan. The key here is to follow a hypnosis session plan that has you listening to dozens of audio sessions every day. This works by helping you lose weight while also altering your mindset so you can learn how to change your eating habits in a way that's permanent.

The most common reason people want to lose weight quickly is because they're about to go on vacation or have an important event and they want a slim figure for the first time in their life. If you want to look slim for a special event or vacation, you should stop worrying about dieting. Instead, focus on exercising more and using stress relief hypnosis sessions while you're at home. If you're going to be outside of the country for many weeks or months, then make a plan to lose weight before you travel.

A study was done where researchers asked 618 overweight people to lose weight by either: eating less and working out more; eating less and doing nothing; exercise with no diet change, eat less and do nothing; or do nothing and eat what they feel like. It was determined that those who did nothing and ate what they felt like lost the least amount of weight. Their weight loss averaged out to less than one pound per week.

The most common reason people struggle with eating healthy is because they are trying to control their food cravings. It's much easier to eat healthy when you learn how to control your food cravings – this is a skill that happens automatically when hypnosis puts you in a trance and alters your mindset for the better. Most people think about food all day long – this leads to them making poor food choices and overeating at night. If you want to lose weight and eat healthy, you should use hypnosis.

Overweight and obese people tend to have a higher level of stress in their lives because of the way they look. It's very common for overweight people to be around other overweight people and they end up feeding off of each other – this leads to more anxiety, which leads to being more stressed, which leads to eating more food. You can change these patterns by using hypnosis while you're at home so you can go on living a normal life while still losing weight.

A lot of men and women struggle with obesity because they have an addictive relationship with food.

There are a number of ways to lose weight but you need to find the right one for you. Weight Loss Hypnosis is an example of a way that may work for some people. The way it works is, a person is put into a state of relaxation and guided to focus on his/her weight issues. The mind and body are calmed so that it is easier to lose weight.

This method seems to be especially effective for people who have a difficult time understanding what they should do in order to lose weight. It can be especially hard for people who have never dieted before, find it difficult to understand the importance of dieting, or lack self-discipline. A person who has tried diets without success may feel overwhelmed at the thought of giving up favorite foods and feeling hungry all the time may sound unpleasant.

Hypnosis helps people see losing weight in a new light. It makes the process less stressful because it teaches a person to accept that giving up favourite foods, for example, is not the end of the world. It also helps people change their reasoning for not losing weight into positive thoughts that will help them lose weight and keep it off. Rather than saying "I don't need to lose weight" hypnosis will help them realize that they want to have more energy and be healthier. This can be just as important to someone as having vanity concerns about their appearance. It is a topic that most people never think about. With so many diets and weight loss foods on the market, it can be hard to know which one is best for you. Weight loss hypnosis may seem like a strange weight loss technique, but it actually does work. It's not uncommon for people who are trying to lose weight (or quit smoking, stop drinking alcohol or drugs) to resist exercise and healthy eating while trying to make these necessary changes in their lives because of the discomfort they experience when faced with limiting their behaviors. This is where hypnosis comes in. The change in eating habits that is required for most people to lose weight and keep it off is just too uncomfortable to be done on willpower alone. If you're not sure that hypnosis can help you lose weight, consider this... no matter what diet you've tried, you never lost the weight permanently . This means that all the diets you've tried have a flaw, an inherent problem with them that prevented permanent weight loss. This is exactly why hypnosis for weight loss works so well -- it bypasses your conscious willpower entirely and addresses the real root of the problem -- your subconscious mind.

#1. Hypnosis for Weight Loss

The unfortunate truth is that most people simply don't understand the psychology behind weight gain and weight loss, so they keep doing the same things that never work. They keep trying to lose weight as quickly as possible, they keep eating processed foods full of artificial ingredients and sugars (which make them hungrier), they keep spending hours on the treadmill instead of playing with their kids. All these behaviors stem from a lack of understanding of what really causes people to gain weight in the first place -- and once they understand that, permanent change becomes inevitable. All it takes is a little hypnosis for weight loss , and you'll finally lose all that excess fat and finally be healthy at a healthy body-weight .

#2. Weight Loss Hypnosis

With weight loss hypnosis, the unconscious mind is made aware of the true cause of your weight gain. The subconscious mind is a lot more effective at processing information than the conscious mind. When you understand why you gained weight in the first place and come to terms with it, you've unlocked a whole new avenue of success in weight-loss. By just being aware of what your body really needs to be healthy, this can be accomplished by hypnosis for weight loss.

#3. Weight Loss Hypnosis - Incredible Results

One of the biggest misconceptions about hypnosis is that it allows people to do things they otherwise wouldn't be able to do. That's true, but in reality, it's more accurate to say that hypnosis enables people to perform the tasks desired by themselves, with ultimate control in their hands. If you really want to lose weight, you can with hypnosis for weight loss. The change in eating habits that is required for most people to lose weight and keep it off is just too uncomfortable to be done on willpower alone. If you're not sure that hypnosis can help you lose weight, consider this -- no matter what diet you've tried, you never lost the weight permanently. This means that all the diets you've tried have a flaw, an inherent problem with them that prevented permanent weight loss. This is exactly why hypnosis for weight loss works so well -- it bypasses your conscious willpower entirely and addresses the real root of the problem -- your subconscious mind.

#4. Hypnosis for Weight Loss - The Science of Sugar Addiction

Sugar addiction is not exactly a new phenomenon, but it's something that needs to be better understood by most Americans. Your brain has a very specific way of regulating how much sugar you take in. When a certain amount of sugar is consumed, your body increases the dopamine levels in your brain which in turn suppresses the production of serotonin. This is how you start to feel "good" when you eat sugar. Well, it's not really good, because it's an addiction and can make you sick. This is why it's so important for people to understand how they feel when they eat something full of sugar. If they understand what sugar does to their brain, they will be able to avoid a future addiction for the sake of their health and happiness.

#5. Hypnosis for Weight Loss - Guided Meditation

With guided meditation, a person is able to learn, understand and change how they feel about themselves. This means that you can think more positively about yourself in order to achieve positive changes in your life. Hypnosis for weight loss is one of those positive changes that can be achieved with guided meditation. There are some who believe it's impossible to lose weight without calories counting or exercising -- these people would be wrong. Hypnosis does not even require you to count calories, and it doesn't require a strict regimented exercise plan -- it actually works better than either of those things would because it helps you attract the right kind of food into your life and avoid the wrong kind altogether.

#6. Hypnosis for Weight Loss - Just Be Happy

Sometimes a person's weight gain is a direct result of emotional issues and not really anything else. Maybe they never ate right in the first place, maybe they were always underweight and now they're just overweight. Whatever the case, weight gain is often a direct result of an emotional issue. It usually has a lot to do with stress and anxiety. Sometimes people just get used to being overweight and can't imagine life any other way -- everything seems so much better that way, even though it's affecting their health negatively. This is where hypnosis for weight loss comes in. If you're feeling stressed or anxious about your weight, hypnosis can help you feel free of those feelings and allow you to be happy.

#7. Hypnosis for Weight Loss - The Power of Intuitive Eating

The main goal of hypnosis for weight loss is to help people learn to eat normally again -- they can stop overeating and eliminate the need to count calories all together. This usually takes place via memory-based sessions that enable the person to see what they were like as a thin person and which foods were most enjoyable when they used to be thin. Then they can be guided through a process that will help them see the foods they were eating before and to identify those foods as being very good for their health.

#8. Hypnosis for Weight Loss - The Basics

The basic steps in hypnosis for weight loss are almost the same as those of any other form of hypnotherapy. The only difference is the way you should be guided by your hypnotherapist. You need to learn how to relax, have a safe and calm environment and use what you learned in other forms of hypnotherapy that don't involve weight loss. You need to be in a relaxed and safe environment with your eyes closed.

#9. Hypnosis for Weight Loss - The Other Grand Rewards of Having a Hypnotist

What is hypnotism and why should you use it? Well, the very first reason is that it can be incredibly effective in helping you lose weight. This is why hypnosis for weight loss makes it over hypnosis for weight loss does so well -- it's because the results are already there without any noticeable effort on your part. This shows that doing hypnosis for weight loss doesn't have to be hard, and that you can just bring yourself to a comfortable place and let the transforming process take its course.

#10. Health Benefits of Hypnosis for Weight Loss

Hypnosis has been proven to help people with a multitude of issues. Most people who have tried hypnosis for weight loss describe it as being one of the most effective self-help strategies they ever discovered. The reason hypnosis is so effective is that it can work on all sorts of people -- young, old, fat, thin, and those that are otherwise in need of a little extra support.

#11. How Hypnosis for Weight Loss Relates to Your Personality

A good hypnotist can help you rebuild your personality and make it much more positive, energetic and focused than before because he is basically changing your perception on life and how you view things in general. You will be able to turn a negative image into a positive one and look at the world with much more positivity.

#12. The History of Hypnosis for Weight Loss

While performing an induction, hypnotherapists are able to connect with people on an emotional level, which is through the release of certain chemicals in the body that activate certain parts of your brain. This allows hypnotists to trigger different feelings, and most people who have tried hypnosis for weight loss say they found it amazingly effective in getting them to feel relaxed enough to initiate the process.

How to Enjoy Healthy Food

Do you feel like you don't enjoy food anymore?

Do you find yourself eating too quickly or wolfing down your food without even tasting it?

Are you always thinking about what's next on your to-do list instead of taking the time to enjoy what's in front of you?

We'll look at how our relationship with healthy foods has changed over time, examine why we often lose our appetite and ability to enjoy good food, and explore some common emotional reasons that make us overeat.

We'll talk about the ways we can use our imagination and memory to help us remember how good healthy food tastes. And, finally, we'll look at some simple strategies that can help you to enjoy a meal again.

Who would have thought that learning to enjoy food again would be so complicated? Now that I've mentioned it, I realize that there are dozens of steps involved in helping yourself learn to enjoy eating healthy foods again. So what are the first steps in your journey back to enjoying food? Here's what I recommend:

1. Start by surrounding yourself with healthy foods—Add colorful fruits and vegetables and other healthy foods to your daily environment.

2. Take a walk—Get out and move around for at least 20 minutes each day.

3. Make friends with your food and learn to enjoy the taste of all foods again!

Step 1: Start by Surrounding Yourself with Healthy Foods

Just as eating junk food is a habit, so is eating healthy foods! Once you begin to choose healthier foods, it will become your new routine. Besides, it's just plain easier to stay on track when healthy foods are readily available. So start by making good choices when it comes to what you keep in your kitchen or how you shop for groceries each week.

Step 2: Take a Walk

When was the last time you took a brisk walk around your neighborhood? Depending on where you live, you may feel like it's not safe to do so alone. If that's the case, have a neighbor with whom you feel comfortable walking regularly.

And if there aren't sidewalks or bike trails in your area, build yourself a "walking trail" by cutting through your neighbors' yards!

If you can't get out and walk regularly, then set a goal to buy yourself some new walking shoes. You won't regret it! Be sure to take regular walks during the day and especially at night. Staying active is one of the best ways to keep off extra pounds.

Step 3: Make Friends with Your Food and Learn to Enjoy the Taste of All Foods Again!

Once you start making better choices, you'll find that it becomes easier and easier to do so. And, essentially, all you have to do is start thinking about good foods differently.

The first step is to imagine and remember how good those foods taste.

Think of a time when you were really hungry and someone offered you a delicious meal with lots of different foods. How many did you eat? You probably ate until you were full, didn't you? Now think back to the last time that happened. Do any negative memories come up for you? You might start thinking about feeling overweight or guilty afterwards. Well, forget that! This is your chance for a fresh start!

Let's pretend that it's right after Thanksgiving dinner. It's a warm, sunny afternoon, and you're taking a walk along the beach. There's a beautiful crystal blue sky with fluffy white clouds and an ocean breeze that just keeps you feeling good.

What kind of foods could you imagine eating? If you have trouble imagining that sort of feast, think about what it would be like to enjoy your favorite types of food again. Look at the list below and write down 5 meals that would be possible for you to enjoy again. Once you've chosen 5 meals, take another look at how to create an imaginary setting in your mind's eye.

Or maybe it would be easier if you were in a movie theater. Picture yourself in the movie theater and write down those foods that you would enjoy as if you were watching a movie. That could also be a great "fantasy" to think about. Whatever kind of setting you choose, make it real and real fun!

Understand? Of course, there are many other options for making friends with your food. You can find some creative ideas on my website, www.discoveringwisdom.com
.

The secret to enjoying good food is simple: It's all the same thing! Think of food as part of your family, and start getting closer to it instead of staying farther away. When you learn to appreciate healthy foods again, you'll be on your way to keeping off unwanted weight and feeling great again!

Why We Lose Our Appetite for Healthy Food

Why are so many of us not enjoying the very food we need the most? Why does good food often look and seem boring compared to some of the "junk" foods we eat? The reason is simple: We've lost our appetite for healthy food. Here are some common reasons why.

It's just too much work!
I used to think that I was a pretty good cook. I made lots of chicken recipes and a few pork recipes, and I usually knew what ingredients were in them. But when I decided to cut out all meat from my diet, I discovered that it was a lot more work than I thought it would be.

I learned that even simple recipes could have ingredients that were hard to pronounce. Just because something is called "turkey" or "steak" doesn't mean that there aren't any other ingredients in the food. Most of us have become accustomed to eating whatever we want whenever we want it, and it is so easy to get into the habit of serving ourselves.

But what happens if you're trying to eat healthy, and it's just not happening? There are a few tricks that can make healthy eating easier on you.

Eat when you get hungry.

When you're used to eating unhealthy foods, your body can get into the habit of craving unhealthy food. When that happens, it's easy to assume that your body really needs those types of foods to keep going all day long. If you're in a situation like this, getting healthy eating back on track can take more willpower than just giving in! I recommend setting a timer for 20-30 minutes away from the table each time you eat something or drink something with calories in it. Understand that your body doesn't need to have another snack right away. It's likely that you can wait until your next meal without giving in to unhealthy cravings. This little trick alone can help you break free from some unhealthy habits like nibbling your way through the day, and it helps you enjoy having a healthy appetite!

Make at least one meal each week a "healthy dinner."

It's really easy to keep eating unhealthy foods because they're everywhere! Fast food restaurants are practically on every street corner these days, and it's nearly impossible not to drive by a pizza place or burger joint when you're driving around town. One way to get around this is to plan ahead for your meals. If you know you're going out with friends or family and they're planning on going to a diner, decide what you'll order ahead of time. If there are fries on the menu, wait until after dinner and have a sensible serving of home-cooked fries. Alternatively, if you plan on eating healthy dinner every week, it's easier to stay away from fast food places when you're out with friends.

Don't use food as a reward.

You may be so used to rewarding yourself with food that it's become part of who you are! If this is the case, it's time to make those changes. Like Jennifer said, you won't feel as good about yourself if you depend on eating unhealthy foods to make you feel better. Instead of rewarding yourself with unhealthy food, reward yourself with the things that make you happy! If you don't want to be involved in unhealthy habits, then don't get involved in them at all!

Don't allow the fact that it will affect your work to keep you from making healthy choices.

One misconception many people have is that eating healthy will cut into their work time and their ability to work out. But this is one of the biggest myths about healthy eating and workouts! Working out actually enhances your ability to work.
I don't always have time to exercise. But I do find that losing weight definitely makes my workout times go more quickly! If you are able to exercise, it's even better because you're actually burning calories while you work out.
You'll also feel better after a workout because it will help you "clear your head." Stress can make us eat more than we should, so it's important to keep it out of the equation! Make sure you are getting enough sleep and eating well so that your body is working at its optimal level!

Do you struggle to enjoy the foods you know are good for you?

Are your cravings for sugary, salty and fatty snacks in the morning, afternoon and evening uncontrollable?

Would you like help taking control of your eating habits, to avoid feeling out of control and bloated all day long?

Hypnosis is a technique that has been around since ancient times. It can be used to help with problems such as weight loss, muscle gain or wound care among others. It has been used for decades to help people improve their lives. It can be used in many ways, from short-term focused goals to permanent life changes.

Many people have difficulties when it comes to eating healthy food. The reason behind this is the same as that of most other addictions: Substitution and reinforcement processes. Eating junk food, you get the satisfaction of appetite and energy, so you eat more of it until you have another craving to satisfy, which again will lead to overeating, overdrinking etc.

When this pattern is repeated enough times it becomes a habit that is hard to break. That's why some people go on strict diets voluntarily for a short amount of time where they only eat one type of fruit or vegetable or fruit-vegetable combinations like grapefruit-carrots or apples-pears. Then after a few days/weeks they suddenly start eating something unhealthy and they find it hard to stop.

At this point, you have become very dependent on the junk food or new food that you've just started to eat. At first, when you are starting to eat healthy food, you may feel deprived of your favorite foods, but in time your taste buds will adapt and new foods will taste amazing (cinnamon-pineapple tarts). This is the main reason why most diets fail: As I have said before, cravings are a big problem if the substitution process is constant. Another reason is that most people start diets on their own initiative, because they want to change something about themselves, and then they think that it's all up to them. They feel like they can't just eat healthy food when they are at a party. On top of that, you don't really know how to deal with the cravings.

This is where hypnosis comes in: It teaches you how to control your impulses and how to enjoy eating healthy food again. So many people have done what you want so badly: To lose weight without having to abandon the foods they love or go on an extreme diet. Hypnosis can help you to enjoy healthy food again, and with a lot of patience and willpower, you can change your eating habits for good.

Let's say that you are the kind of person who always has a piece of cake or a treat at every occasion when invited to a party. You eat it because you feel like it and not because it is better for you. You eat too much chocolate, alcohol or some other junk food that contains fat, sugar or salt in large quantities. Sooner or later, you will end up with cravings: You want your cake (or your chocolate bar etc.) so much that you just have to acquire it. But then you eat it and you are full of cravings again, so you go to the kitchen and eat something else. Then, when that's over, you probably feel guilty about eating too much and you start to think about how bad your diet is. So what do you do? You go out for a walk, jog or whatever activity involves exercise. This will help burn off some of the calories (and will also make you feel better than before). But at the same time it acts as a reinforcement: You are now doing something healthy for yourself physically and mentally (feeling better about yourself). And now there is another craving that needs to be satisfied: The desire to eat healthy food again. You need to go and buy yourself more healthy food. And then you feel bad because you could have just bought yourself the junk food, but you are always full of health problems. So now you start thinking about going to the doctor for help. But, in hypnosis, we can teach you how to deal with your cravings and your impulses more effectively.

How does it work?

Hypnosis works by replacing unhealthy habits with healthier ones that are guided by a therapist or dietitians who follow a specific diet plan tailored to each client's needs. By following this plan, the client is no longer dependent on eating healthier foods or avoiding those that they enjoy. Hypnosis can teach people how to enjoy healthy food again by restoring the taste buds to like them once again. The cravings and urges to eat unhealthy foods disappear.

You will feel more satisfied with healthier foods: Hypnosis does not replace healthy eating with dieting, but puts the focus on eating less quantity but more variety of food choices, you will naturally eat better and not completely abandon your favorite foods.

In hypnosis, you will learn to deal with your cravings more effectively: Cravings are one of the most common problems when it comes to dieting. But the difference between a craving and truly enjoying food is that cravings never increase in intensity. So, while you crave for something sweet, it is possible to consume something sweet like a piece of chocolate and then feel like you are satisfied with what you have eaten. But if it's an extremely strong craving, then it can lead to obesity or binge eating disorder – which is considered an addiction by many psychologists. This is why hypnosis helps you not only with the physical side of food addiction but also with how we as humans are wired. Through hypnosis, you will learn how to deal with your cravings.

But you need to do your part, too: I have trained many people with hypnosis and they are all very motivated to lose weight, which is a good start. But even though they learn to deal with their cravings, if they still eat the same foods and eat them in the same quantities as before, it will be difficult for them to lose weight or change their eating habits for good. That's why you need willpower and patience: Some things will happen naturally over time and others take some effort on your part. I want you to be prepared for that so that your hypnosis sessions will be more successful. It's not the end of the world if you have a craving for cake when your hypnosis session ends. If you have your own goal that you want to reach, then you will find it in the course of time.

Hypnotherapy is not just for weight loss: Many people come into my office thinking that they've tried everything else and are looking for a quick fix in order to lose weight. It's true that losing weight requires discipline and determination, but it doesn't have to be the only goal for every single client. You may need therapy for other reasons as well: I often see clients struggling with issues like stress, anxiety or depression. And I have helped many of them by putting them into a deep state of relaxation where they can find answers on their own. I want you to be open to the possibility that hypnotherapy might help you in ways that are not directly connected to your weight loss. It's not all about losing weight – it's about helping you find inner peace, too. You might benefit from hypnosis even if you are not overweight or planning on losing weight.

How to enjoy healthy food and still lose weight? The answer might have been found with a study by Tulane University. In the study participants who ate an all-you-can-eat buffet and listened to hypnosis lost more weight than those in the control group.

Some people have used hypnosis to transform their lives, imagine what it could do for you? You may feel like your struggles are insurmountable, but they don't need to be with these changes right here and now. That's not all though! Here are some other ways that hypnosis can help you stay informed of what happens while you sleep and aid in relieving stress or pain.

Many people choose to use hypnosis to combat their specific problem areas. The weight loss industry is filled with countless numbers of options to try, but very few of them are truly effective. We have your best interest at heart and stand behind every one of our programs because we are confident that you will achieve your goals.

Most people know that following a healthy, balanced diet is important to their well-being. Yet for some, living a full and enjoyable life seems next to impossible with all the guilt and shame associated with food choices. With the power of hypnosis, you can be happy in your body, enjoy what you eat without feeling guilty and be confident in your choice of lifestyle.

Do you love having all the comforts of your home, but still want to go out with friends and enjoy a night out on the town? With self-hypnosis, you have the best of both worlds. You can simply relax your way through a busy day and allow the rest of it to go by without noticing. Then when you're ready to feel energized and alive again, just close your eyes and get what you need within moments.

Techniques to Reduce Food Intake and Food Craving

Techniques to reduce food intake and reduce cravings have been developed and must be integrated into any weight loss plan for sustainable success. Hypnosis has been found to be a successful way to reduce food intake and cravings by creating a neural connection between feelings of hunger and taste with feelings of fullness and satiety. This is accomplished through eating mindfully, which involves paying attention to the experience of eating. This promotes greater enjoyment of meals, allows one to delay gratification, reduces the number of calories consumed during the meal, helps one practice portion control, enables one to better recognize hunger cues before they become overwhelming, as well as gains in satisfaction from healthy eating habits.

Hypnosis can also be used to create a positive neural connection between food and feelings of fullness, and between food and feelings of satiety. This helps to reduce cravings associated with the consumption of unhealthy foods, which helps improve one's food intake as well. Hypnosis can be very effective in helping you not only understand why you overeat, especially in response to emotional triggers or cues, but it can also help you develop a greater control over those urges.

The Control-Override Scale Model is an effective means for increasing self-control by providing positive encouragement to take better control of unhealthy urges that result from an overeating episode or bingeing behaviors. Eating mindfully and controlling urges can be reinforced by using guided imagery of very desirable outcomes that will result from your mindful eating and control-override behavior. These very desirable outcomes are visualized in the form of a movie that contains positive affirmation, representations of self-control, and affective images that correspond to the emotions you want to experience after bingeing or overeating. By visualizing these positive experiences over and over again, one creates an effective neural connection between the act of overeating and feelings of satiety. This can decrease the occurrence of binge eating as well as lead to weight loss.

Other techniques for reducing food intake include using self-hypnosis to trigger feelings of fullness when eating an appropriate sized meal. The fullness feelings trigger the development of a positive association between eating and satiety. This can be enhanced by using self-hypnosis to remind oneself that if one were to eat more than one's daily amount, there would probably be feelings of discomfort.

This is done by using a "savoring technique" in which you are reminded that you can take longer to finish your meal, and that even if you did eat more than your daily predetermined portion, a full feeling would eventually occur. You then take small bites of your food with full attention paid to the food itself and its taste and texture. When you have finished eating, you experience how empty it feels.

It is a good idea to be aware of one's hunger and fullness cues before eating. If you are eating a meal that includes fats or sweets, it is important to eat slowly and mindfully, focusing on the food as if it were a treat.

It is also important to be aware of your feelings at higher levels of fullness or satiety. It is sometimes better not to overeat especially in response to emotional cues because this often leads to feelings of discomfort after the meal has been consumed. For instance, if you are at a party with friends and want to eat everything offered, you may suffer from stomach cramps later on when the food is digested.

If you experience stress, you are more likely to eat in response to stress-induced cues as a form of comfort. By using self-hypnosis to relax, one can help diminish the stress-triggers that cause eating binges as a way of coping with anxiety. By becoming aware of your feelings and the real reasons for your emotional eating, distraction techniques can be used effectively to stop yourself from overeating. You can increase awareness by practicing self-hypnosis and mindfulness meditation. This helps you get in touch with emotions that cause desire to relieve them with food intake. Furthermore, it helps recognize satiety signals while eating and feel more satisfied after eating an appropriate sized meal.

Guided imagery can also be used effectively to develop a positive association between food and feeling full or satiated. This is done by imagining the last meal enjoyed in a pleasant and enjoyable experience. You imagine yourself eating slowly, savoring each bite, enjoying the way the food tastes, smells and feels in your mouth. It is important not to think about other things while eating this way because it can slow down digestion and lead to feelings of discomfort after overeating. If one regularly uses this guided imagery technique before eating, it can help trigger feelings of fullness when eating an appropriate sized meal. This can decrease cravings for unhealthy foods as well as help one develop healthy eating habits that result in weight loss success.

Other methods for inducing a positive feedback loop in connection with positive feelings, healthy eating and weight management include the use of virtual reality. This involves using machines that project images into one's brain while one is concentrating on visualizing something pleasant. Additionally, it is a good idea to stick to small portions of food at mealtimes so that no portion is overeaten and the result is a full feeling. This correlates with having an effective control-override behavior and also helps to create a positive association between food and satiety.

In addition, it is useful to understand why or when we overeat or binge eat by understanding our feeding patterns. For example, many people use food to sooth themselves when they are feeling down. For this reason, it is important to recognize the emotional and situational variables associated with eating binges and binge eating.

Another method that has been shown to be effective for reducing binge eating is the use of sensory interventions such as food diaries. In this case, one keeps track of a diet and pattern of eating in a form that promotes self-honesty without triggering emotionally-induced overeating. The idea behind this technique is that by recording what we eat daily or at least on a weekly basis, we are able to see how much we are actually consuming in relation to our caloric needs. This process enables one to make a self-directed plan that will help them attain their goals.

Hypnosis and Weight Management Success

Depending on the particular individual, hypnosis may play a role in helping them lose weight. Some people find hypnosis to be helpful; others do not have as much success with it as they expected. Most people do not see good results from hypnosis until after their basic needs are met. Not everyone is open to this form of treatment either -- some believe in it and others do not without ever trying it first. As with any form of weight loss, it is important for one to understand the possible benefits and risks of hypnosis as an effective weight loss tool.

Hypnosis is a stress-reducing form of therapy that can reduce eating behavior problems. A person who is hypnotized can learn how to use various techniques learned through work with a doctor or therapist in order to stop binge eating from interfering with daily life. This can include adopting positive, healthy eating habits and weight management techniques as well as learning to identify and eliminate negative or destructive thoughts that may surround overeating.

The use of hypnosis as a way of removing excess weight is not unreasonable when used in addition to other more common weight loss techniques. Hypnosis can be used for the following purposes:

As a method of improving one's self-esteem, self-image, and self-confidence by helping them see themselves in a new light. This can be achieved by performing actions that one is not accustomed to doing such as standing up straight or talking to strangers. By doing this, they force themselves to change their negative behavior (slouching, being shy) and replace it with a more positive self image (standing tall, feeling less inhibited). As a way of helping one to identify and eliminate negative behaviors such as eating when they feel that they are not hungry or having unrealistic emotional responses about losing weight. This can be achieved through identifying and eliminating distressing thoughts that may be able to lead to eating excessively or is being a negative regulator of normal eating behavior, such as telling oneself that one is never going to lose weight or that only disasters will happen because you are overweight.

Just like in any other form of hypnotherapy, the results from this type of therapy can vary depending on the practitioner. The practitioner may guide their patient through different aspects of the hypnosis, while the patient maintains control over themselves and their breathing. It is also important for the patient to be able to stay in control of their own mind. If they are constantly responding to suggestions in a way that the practitioner has not intended, then this may result in undesirable side effects. Therefore, it is very important that the patient should be motivated and understand that motivation helps them achieve positive results with hypnotherapy.

It is not entirely clear how much weight people can expect to lose from doing CORE hypnotherapy sessions, but it seems like a very achievable goal if motivation and self-control are at their best. It is good to note that there are several people who have succeeded with this type of therapy, both male and female alike.

As with any form of therapy for weight loss, one must be mindful of the possible side effects. They include fatigue after a session or 2, headache, minor anxiety that does not interfere with daily life and no one knows how much weight will be lost. Although these side effects might occur they are usually temporary and end when the problem is solved. One may lose weight and keep it off without having to repeat sessions or undergo medical procedures if under hypnosis and still working on achieving their goals.

The benefits of hypnosis as a means of managing one's eating behavior are found to be effective in decreasing binge eating behavior. Although it is highly recommended that one consult a physician for any form of therapy, CORE hypnotherapy has proved to be effective in helping one to achieve healthy eating habits and weight management.

Some people are afraid of the effects that hypnosis may have on them, but hypnosis does not cause long-term mental or physical problems. A person who is hypnotized can learn how to use various techniques learned through work with a doctor or therapist in order to stop binge eating from interfering with their daily life. This can include adopting positive, healthy eating habits and weight management techniques as well as learning to identify and eliminate negative or destructive thoughts that may surround overeating.

As with any form of therapy for weight loss, it is important to consult a physician before trying this form of therapy. Hypnotists are also encouraged to verify that the patient understands and agrees with the information they are telling them. CORE hypnotherapy has proven to be effective in helping one lose weight by bringing out the positive aspects of their personality and helping them overcome negative eating habits such as binge eating, excessive eating or emotional eating. If performed alone, this form of therapy can be used in conjunction with other forms of weight loss therapy or counseling in order to bring out even more positive effects.

It is suggested that one does not use hypnosis as a way of changing one's personality as this may result in negative side effects such as changes in behavior and personality. Hypnotists should only provide suggestions for how the patient should alter their lifestyle or behavior that they are already following. If these don't help, then the therapist may suggest other forms of therapy to help this individual change their eating behaviors.

It is important to understand that the initial results from CORE hypnotherapy sessions may seem minimal to those who have never tried it, but over time this positive approach will take hold and bring even more success for those who are open to it. Unlike other forms of therapy for weight loss, hypnosis is believed to have no side effects. This form of therapy can be used in conjunction with other treatments or programs and it can also help the individual concerned eliminate their cravings for high calorie foods which may result in overeating. When this happens, the individual may be able to lose weight and keep it off without having to repeat sessions or undergo medical procedures.

The final outcome that you get from hypnotherapy will depend on how much effort you put into it and whether you are willing to give up some of your bad eating habits. Some people are afraid to use hypnosis because they believe that it is dangerous and will cause psychological damage. This belief is not valid as much of what the person may do or say under hypnosis is what they already want to do or say. Some people will go into a deeper state of relaxation depending on their level of relaxation when they are hypnotized. For instance, some people have a high threshold for deep relaxation while others have a low threshold which makes them go into deeper states of relaxation and may lead to mental disturbances.

If you are contemplating using hypnosis as a form of therapy, it is advisable that you plan ahead before calling a hypnotist, Before you call a hypnotist, you must ensure that the person has relevant experience in the field and that they are fully certified. As with any form of therapy, it is advisable to seek a second opinion in order to obtain treatment for binge eating because this form of therapy is not always successful. However, if you are open to it and enjoy the experience, it may work wonders for your weight loss goals. Hypnosis is a highly effective way to lose weight when used as part of a comprehensive treatment plan. This includes hypnosis sessions that are performed by a trained professional who has been certified with the National Guild of Hypnotists or other organizations. The following is a list of the various positive effects of hypnosis: Weight loss due to a reduction in calories consumed.

Role playing coping skills help soothe anxiety and negative emotions.

Helping one to form new habits which will help them lose weight and change eating behavior such as limiting the amount of food that they eat or sticking to healthy eating habits.

Hypnosis can be a helpful tool when used in conjunction with other forms of therapy for weight loss. Most hypnotists will guide their patient through different aspects of the hypnosis, while the patient maintains control over themselves and their breathing. It is also important for the patient to be able to stay in control of their own mind. If they are constantly responding to suggestions in a way that the hypnotist has not intended, this may result in undesirable side effects. Therefore it is very important that the patient should be motivated and understand that motivation helps them achieve positive results with hypnotherapy.

Do not be afraid of using hypnosis as a form of treatment for obesity and make sure that you are getting the best advice. This will help you to avoid unnecessary side effects and give you the opportunity to use this form of therapy as a way of losing weight. Although it is highly recommended that one consult a physician for any form of therapy, CORE hypnotherapy has proved to be effective in helping one to achieve healthy eating habits and weight management.

How to Overcome Portion Control and Overeating Difficulties?

One of the most commonly cited reasons for weight gain is that people eat too much or eat things they should not. These are behaviors that can be difficult to change because they are often habitual, but there are many ways to work on breaking this habit and eating more mindfully.

Sometimes, an eating problem is due to a physical problem such as gastric bypass surgery or the need for a medication that results in the loss of appetite. If you are suffering from not being able to eat enough, you may benefit from hypnotherapy to see if this can help you with your eating issues. If you have to take a medication that makes you nauseous or lose your appetite, hypnosis can help you get through that time. If you have gastric bypass surgery, hypnosis can help with the changes you need to make in how your body digests food. Some people will find that they can eat more after the surgery.

Many times overeating is a problem, not because people are eating too much food, but because they are not eating in the proper way. Many people eat with their eyes instead of their mind and this can lead to overeating. Other times, they may be consuming things that do not agree with them and this can cause diarrhea or other issues. In these situations, hypnosis can help with weight loss based on how body processes food.

Some people may fail to eat when they should or generally in
wrong foods for them. This can lead to poor health
such as depression and anxiety attacks an
through hypnotherapy, including wei

OLI

One of the most common issues for people today is eating too much and eating the wrong foods. There are many reasons this happens, both physical and mental, but it is important to make sure you know why you are not able to eat more in a healthy way. The reason behind this behavior can often be determined with hypnotherapy. This could include gastric bypass surgery or other reasons that make it difficult for people to eat more foods that they want.

Are you struggling with being able to control your eating? Do you have difficulties controlling your cravings for food that is not necessarily good for you? Have you been ignoring your body's signals that it's full?

"Portion distortion" is a major part of the problem. The average portion sizes have tripled over the past fifty years. There are a lot of reasons why we have this gigantic issue, but the most important thing to do about this is to know what kind of portions are appropriate for you and your diet and then stick to them.

Understanding Portion Sizes

Most people don't really know how many calories they are consuming or the true amount of food that they eat in general. Portion control should be taught as early in life as possible, but there's no reason why anyone can't learn it at any age.

Some people can have trouble figuring out what a healthy portion size is. The best way to know is by reading the nutritional labels on your food and then stick to it. If you are confused, ask a nutritionist or a doctor to help you.

A Healthy Portion Is the Right Amount of Food for Your Body

Research has shown that "the best way to eat" is to keep track of what you are eating and make sure that it complements your body's functions well. Most people don't need to eat more food than they need because there is a widely available surplus of food in the market. It's simply not necessary to be overweight.

There are a lot of unnecessary calories in the average diet with this growing portion sizes. If you want to lose weight, then you should go on a diet that has low calorie consumption and a moderate intake of healthy foods. That's what I recommend for everyone who wants to lose weight, but it is important that you know your body and learn how much food you truly need in order to be healthy.

Weight loss and control of overeating is one of the most common issues people face. In America, for example, the Centers for Disease Control and Prevention estimates that 69% of adults are overweight or obese. Problems with overeating can not only lead to weight gain and health problems but can also lead to depression when you cannot control your unhealthy eating habits.

Hypertension Scales

The first step is getting an accurate reading on your current weight using a hypertension scale. Hypertension scales should be calibrated periodically to ensure accuracy. This will provide a baseline for understanding changes in your weight over time so you know if you are meeting your goals or sustaining any success in weight loss measures over time.

BMI

Obesity is defined by a BMI reading that is greater than 30. BMI stands for body mass index, and it is a measurement of your current weight in relation to your height. This reading helps to determine your healthy weight range and provides information on how much you should weigh.

Calories Burned with Exercise

The key to overcoming overeating and improving weight loss efforts is dieting activities along with exercise. Calculating the calories burned during exercise can be useful when planning a diet or caloric intake needs for the day, week, or month. The amount of calories burned will vary depending on the intensity of exercise activities as well as the duration and type of activity.

This post will help you with:

- How to overcome emotional feelings that could trigger overeating
- How to reduce your appetite or cravings
- Learn about the power of hypnosis and explore how this could help you lose weight
- Help you identify specific goals and weight loss targets
- Thoroughly explain how appetite blockers can be used in conjunction with a healthy lifestyle

Do you find yourself overeating and eating things you don't even like? Are you someone who needs a certain amount of food to feel satisfied? Do you ever feel like your just going to keep eating until you die? Are there times when the idea of cooking for yourself sounds so overwhelming that it's easier just to get something fast at the drive-through window, or out at the restaurant, even when it's not something healthy for your body? Do you feel like overeating since your teens, all through out your 20s? Does the idea of dieting make you feel like a failure or even hopeless? Do you find yourself eating things that are not optimal for your body and have no nutritional value?

First of all, I want to share some things about me. I have been hypnosis for 3 years now and I have used hypnosis with more than 300 people. They have had a range of issues from weight issues, pre-diabetes, diabetes, depression and anxiety to sky-high blood pressure! I specialize in weight loss using hypnosis.

Weight loss is difficult because it is a complex issue. It's not simply about calories in and calories out. All our brains and bodies are driven by emotion, past emotional issues that we didn't deal with and addictions develop in our lives. There are also physical issues that can lead to weight gain such as being overweight, having high blood pressure or cholesterol.

Emotional Issues: For some people the idea of dieting makes them feel like failure or hopeless or they worry about the looks of people at work or school. They might have experienced family conflicts over weight issues in their past (see more below about how a hypnotherapist can help with these). Some people's weight issues are tied to how they were treated growing up. For example, blame might be placed on the person who is overweight blaming themselves and not having any self-worth. The belief that you are not good enough or that you can't do anything right could also lead to overeating patterns to cope with these feelings. These patterns can start very early in life and the brain has no way of differentiating between then and now.

Emotional Eating: People can be driven to overeat by emotions that they aren't aware of. Emotions are all around us and we are constantly experiencing them. The full name of emotional eating is "unconscious eating". It's easy to identify our physical hunger when we feel it in our stomachs, but so many times emotional hunger can take place without you knowing it, yet a lack of these feelings could be the reason you eat too much or not enough food at meal times.

If any of these statements ring true to some degree, then hypnosis may be able to help. Hypnosis is an amazing tool for making long lasting changes in your life. It can help you overcome weight issues, improve performance at work, help you develop a healthy relationship with food, and much more. In this chapter I'll talk about how to use hypnosis for weight loss, but this chapter is also valuable for anyone trying to improve their health in general.

Hypnosis helps by giving you the ability to identify what it is that sets off your eating behavior and also encouraging you to change how you think about food. Over years of experience, I have learned which thoughts will stop someone from overeating and which thoughts will increase consumption habits. The former includes thoughts like "If I eat now, I'll never be hungry again." The latter includes thoughts like "There is no point in starting until I have finished."

This is a tool I have used with hundreds of people, and it is always helpful. It works on the subconscious level and takes no extra effort or action from you. For the most part you will not even realize you are doing it.

Hypnosis isn't going to make your weight disappear on its own. However, it can help you get more control over your eating habits and dieting process. This cahpter will talk about what hypnosis can do for weight loss but it's also very useful for those who need help with their diets in general, as well as those that want to change their attitudes towards food.

It doesn't matter what type of diet you are following, or if you have been following a diet and not losing weight. It doesn't matter how much you weigh right now, or if you are just trying to lose a few pounds or even more than a hundred pounds.

Hypnosis is going to allow you to change how your think about food and the portions that you eat. After that it will allow you to change how your body reacts to food, so it's easier for you to know when your full and stop eating before consuming too much.

I have helped people lose weight with hypnosis alone, but this is rare. Most people will need to follow a diet and a workout plan as well in order for this to work. You should not expect hypnosis to be able to make you lose weight overnight, or even with just one session. That's not how it works, though there are things you can do right away that will also assist your weight loss.

Benefits of Hypnosis

So, what exactly is hypnosis? Is it something that I am talking about? How do I know if it is working? Is it real or just fantasy? If this is something new for you, then let me give you a little background information to help explain what exactly hypnosis is. First off, let me share with you the definition from Dictionary.com – "a hypnotic state induced by guiding suggestions of the hypnotist; deep trance."

So, in a nutshell, hypnosis is just a type of trance that you can go into so you can make changes in your life. When you are in a trance, your mind is quiet, and it is receptive to the suggestions that are given to you. It means that while you are in this sleep like state, anything and everything can be suggested to your subconscious mind. I am not saying that this is an easy thing to do or something that everyone can do naturally. It does require practice and study, but most people find it far easier than they expected once they start practicing it on themselves.

How You Become Hypnotized

Before you ever decide to learn hypnosis, you will need to get past the fear of it. As I talked about earlier, that is the number one reason why people do not want to try this out, so you will need to understand that it is something they can learn how to do. You may be afraid of finding out that hypnosis is a fraud. You may be afraid that it will make you go crazy or even put you in a coma if you even try and use it without proper training. If that sounds like you, then fear not my friend. You can get over this fear and start learning hypnosis without ever having to experience any of those things.

If you want to learn hypnosis just for fun, then you are going to have to get past the need for any form of proof that your work is actually helping people in any way. Even though there is not a single form of proof that it ever did work before, I am willing to bet that has also been the case on all the other parts of your life as well. This is how life works – we do everything because we want something good or bad out of it and we choose to believe that our actions will bring about those results in some way.

Hypnosis isn't any different. Even though you will not be able to predict the results of your actions, you can still choose to start learning hypnosis. The best way to do this is by trying it out. You will have to get past the first initial sessions when you might not achieve anything or even fall asleep. That said, if you really want to make a change in your life and learn a new skill that is going to help improve your overall health and well-being, then hypnosis is definitely worth a try. If nothing else, at least it's better than watching tv or reading books all day long.

Common Obstacles in Diet

One of the difficulties faced by those who are obese comes from finding energy to maintain their workouts. Being overweight can make some people feel tired very easily due to being overweight causing them to breathe harder and faster when they do any sort of physical activity. This can make it hard for the person to get inspired to continue with their workouts.

It is also true that those who are overweight, due to their weight, are more prone to feeling sluggish and less interested in performing physical activity because of being in pain. Oftentimes, being overweight can cause several health problems like heart disease, which can make physical activities uncomfortable and less enjoyable for them.

Researchers have proven that being obese can cause difficulty in performing simple daily tasks like walking or climbing the stairs without gasping for breath or even pain on their knees or hips. Because of this, they may feel less motivated to exercise freely and sometimes skip workouts altogether.

One of the common problems for those who are obese is losing control over eating and overeating. Those who are unable to control their hunger or appetite may have too much cravings for food, which sometimes lead to them eating more than they normally would consume daily. This can lead to gaining extra weight and making it harder for the person to lose weight.

Some obese people also have difficulties performing physical activities due to their weight which suggest that they often take a day off from exercising because of pain or discomfort during workouts. As a result of ending their workouts, this can make it difficult for the person to lose weight in a healthy and healthy way.

It's no secret: dieting is hard. Eating healthy and exercising are two of the most common resolutions made by people after their new year when coming up with self-improvement goals. It's also no secret that people don't always succeed in these resolutions... For this reason, a lot of resources devoted to weight loss are often focused on motivation and encouragement rather than pure knowledge. Weight loss hypnosis, guided meditation, and gastric band hypnosis, in contrast, focus more on your subconscious mind (or "unconscious," as it's sometimes called) to change what you're thinking or feeling about food and changing your relationship with it.

When dieting is driven by peer pressure, which it often is in our society, and fad diets that tend to fail quickly and for the most part don't offer a long-term solution, certain things can be overlooked. For example, many different foods that you could eat to make you thinner are often overlooked. Many less healthy foods - ones that are high in calories but low in nutrients - are also often overlooked while dieting. The question then becomes: What exactly is people trying to lose weight? From a purely physical standpoint, what does being on a diet consist of?

The answer: dieting consists of burning off more calories than you take in. This process is known as "calorie restriction," and it's the best way to lose weight. Many people choose to do this by skipping meals or cutting out certain foods from their diets, but this is often the most ineffective way to go about it. In this chapter, I will explain why you should cut out certain foods from your diet while on a weight loss diet and how you can do so safely.

These days, more and more people are turning to hypnosis as a way to lose weight. While you may not be familiar with what hypnosis is or how it works, you've probably heard of some of the benefits that people experience when they undergo hypnosis. But when it comes to weight loss...

The idea of "mindfulness," often associated with certain parts of Eastern religions like Buddhism, is becoming more and more popular in Western society. The entire point of this approach to eating is to be as aware as possible of your body and how much you're eating at every meal. This is done by literally sitting down at each meal, being mindful, and counting each portion. That's right - counting how many bites you take!

One of the reasons why so many people wind up with bad eating habits is because they're so used to just mindlessly throwing food into their mouths. It's just become a habit after all these years, and they don't realize how much they are actually eating until it's too late. Mindfulness helps you to realize exactly how much you're eating at every meal, but not only that:

Need motivation for weight loss? Need someone to push you towards your goal of being thin? The best way to lose weight and stay with it is by overcoming the excuses that prevent you from achieving your goals. Do you want to know the excuses that prevent people from losing weight and some techniques that will help you to overcome them?

Sometimes called "silent" or "inner" voices, your self-talk is probably one of the main reasons why you fail at achieving your goals. It can be a very powerful force, either helping you succeed or pushing you into failure. Learning how to control your thoughts is an essential part of any weight loss program.

For many people, controlling their thoughts leads to greater success in dieting by helping them stay focused on their goals. When fat loss is your goal, you will lose weight. But in order to succeed, you have to control your thoughts and stop yourself from thinking negative thoughts. If you can do this, then you'll be able to build confidence through willpower.

On the other hand, if you're not able to control your self-talk, this can easily lead to feelings of guilt and failure that will prevent you from achieving any progress in your weight loss.

In a world where everyone seems to be focused on diets and dieting, it's easy for a person to get lost and confused about what the best diet for them is really like in the beginning stages. Dieting can be a very difficult process to go through: you're cutting out sweets, toast, and other foods that you enjoy every day. It's easy to get tired of this and think of all the meals that you can no longer eat anymore.

But what people don't realize is that there are so many different types of dieting options out there. And not only that but depending on your personal goals and expectations for yourself, the best diet for you might actually vary. For example, if your goal is to lose weight, then the best diet for you might be a low-calorie diet. However, if your goal is to become healthy and fit, then a low calorie diet might not be the best choice.

It's important to remember that there are many different types of diets out there:

A low carbohydrate diet or keto diet is when your carbohydrate intake is very minimal. The main focus of this kind of dieting program is on eating fat and protein rich meals instead of carbs.

Everyone has a story about their struggles with dieting - everything from why they can't seem to keep the weight off, to what just doesn't agree with their body. There are a number of factors that contribute to these difficulties - including hypnosis, guided meditation, and gastric band hypnosis. The reason is that when we're tempted with food, our brain takes in all the sensory information about the tempting food in an effort to determine if it's a good idea to eat it. Sometimes this makes us want to eat even though we know we should not do so. The hypnosis and guided meditation sessions that are included in this weight loss program will help you change your brain's automatic response to those tempting foods. Even if you feel you must eat everything in sight to stick to your diet, you can break this habit. By giving the brain a different response, you can help your weight loss succeed.

The biggest obstacle to being able to lose weight is the idea that "you can't eat just anything." It's true - you can't. But what you can do is pick out a few small, healthy snacks and work your way up from there. And while it's impossible to eat just one or two healthy snacks at a time, it's possible to work toward eating more and more of them.

Most people know they shouldn't eat just any old junk food to lose weight. What they don't know is that you can't lose weight by eating "just any old junk food" as well. There are certain foods that are permitted when you're dieting and there are certain foods that should be avoided. But in addition to the actual food itself, there's the idea of being able to eat it as well...

In many cases, people who struggle with their weight don't really know everything they should or can do about it. This is why it's not uncommon for someone to find themselves in a vicious cycle: Eating healthy helps me feel and look better - but I end up gaining weight because of it! It's a shame - but people just don't know how to break out of this seemingly endless loop...

Too often, people think that they must change everything all at once when they start a diet. They try to make every meal a salad, cut out all snacks, and tell themselves that they'll only eat this one food or that one food. It's hard enough to do this when you're losing weight - imagine how it feels when the weight just doesn't seem to be coming off anymore!

The program we have available for you provides a short, guided meditation session which helps get your mind clear and focused on your goal; it also provides hypnosis sessions which aim to help reinforce the improvements that are being made during the guided meditation session. The program is designed in such a way that your goal is achieved at a pace that's comfortable for you.

We like to think of weight loss as a journey into a healthier you, and we know that it can require discipline. But for those who are willing to take the first step, our hypnosis program is here to help. Here at HypnosisForWeightLoss.com we know that weight loss is something that anyone can achieve - even if you have struggled in the past - so whether you're looking to shed a few extra pounds or get them off permanently, we're here to help...

Many of us do not have an eating disorder but are still unhappy with our body image. We weigh ourselves every day and obsess over numbers on a scale. That's why we've created a program that teaches you how to change your relationship with food and is not based on "dieting" or restricting things in your diet that you love. By using this program, you will learn the tools you need to make lasting changes with your weight - changes that will stick even when the weight loss is over...

Most of us are familiar with the idea of "weight loss." If we're not in shape, we want to lose weight; if we are overweight, we want to lose even more. Weight loss can be difficult to accomplish though because it's so easy to get off track when trying to shed some pounds - especially if there is no help or guidance available...

If you've struggled with your weight for some time and would like to know how to lose weight by eating more healthy foods, our program is designed to help you make lasting changes. It's based on a series of guided meditations which use hypnosis to help you focus on the goal you're trying to achieve. The changes made by the program are designed in such a way that they can stay with you even when weight loss ends...

Many people think that losing weight is easy - all they have to do is get in shape and watch the pounds melt away. And while this may work for some people, it doesn't work for everyone - especially those who have already tried dieting and worked hard but failed in the past.

Dieting Motivation

Why do people pursue dieting? It's a complex issue, with several factors that can make or break dieting relationships. To keep this review focused on why hypnosis is useful in losing weight, it's important to understand what motivates people who work hard to accomplish weight loss goals. There are certainly several reasons why individuals choose to eat healthy foods and exercise regularly - but there are also many reasons for not doing so. Hypnotic techniques help you gain insight into what truly motivates you to eat right and move your body - whether it is healthy for you or not. For some people, the idea of dieting or exercise is enough to make them avoid these behaviors. But for others, it needs to be done for a reason. When we're in a hypnotic trance and given suggestions about what we should or shouldn't do - our body reacts accordingly - but you can learn why this happens and change your habits accordingly.

Dieting With Hypnosis

When you've tried every diet on the book, it's time to seek professional help for your weight loss goals. You may have been told that it's impossible to lose weight with hypnosis or guided meditation, but this is not true. You can reach your weight loss goals with the right combination of hypnosis and guided meditation. If you would like to try out these methods, there is one thing you need to remember - and that is that it's absolutely essential to be in a hypnotic trance during these sessions. Even if you just listen to the tapes, it's not going to work when you're thinking about what you should or shouldn't do during the exercise. Also, people for whom hypnosis doesn't work well may want to consider using hypnosis and guided meditation together. The combination of these two methods can be very powerful when used properly - and will often lead to positive results sooner than either technique would on its own.

Dieting With Hypnosis and Guided Meditation

Combining hypnosis and guided meditation is a powerful way to overcome your weight loss hurdles. You may be wondering what guided meditation is, and how it's different from other types of methods. It's true that there are many methods of losing weight - but the most successful of these are the long-term ones that you incorporate into your lifestyle. The key to this type of dieting is in the change in behavior - which our minds respond to as if it were a result of our unique physiology. This is why hypnosis is so useful as an aid for permanent behavioral change - since your mind will interpret all input (in this case from hypnosis) using its own filter.

How to Do Exercise and How to Find Motivation

These questions are very common nowadays. But what if there is a way to get rid of all your troubles, without even moving an inch?

Hypnosis is the induction of a trance-like state in order to achieve a heightened state of intellectual or emotional functioning. Using hypnosis for weight loss, this means going into a trance and visualizing eating less food than you normally would and exercising more. Hypnosis can also be used for gastric band hyposis—this is when the mind believes it has been fitted with an artificial stomach, which makes appetite suppression easier.

How can you hypnotize yourself and lose weight?

The key to self-hypnosis is to always be calm and relaxed. If you are stressed, it will be harder to slip into a state of deep relaxation. So here are some useful tips that will help you relax before you begin your hypnosis techniques for weight loss:

• Lie down on the couch or bed, with pillows supporting your neck and head. You should be lying flat with your feet on the ground, knees bent at a 90 degree angle and hands by your side, palms facing up. This is similar to the position babies sleep in; it's called the "fetal position.

• Close your eyes and take 10 deep, slow breaths by counting your breaths from 1 to 10.

• Start to count your breathing in a monotone voice. After each inhale, count '1', after each exhale, count either '2' or '3'.

When you reach a total of 10 breaths, open your eyes. You should have been able to focus on the counting sound in your ears rather than the outside world. If not, try counting thoughts or repeating a word over and over until you are comfortable focusing on it. The point is to try focusing as narrowly as you can to make it easier for yourself to relax further.

How to do hypnosis for weight loss?

Hypnosis is a techniques that works by changing your subconscious. You achieve this state through a combination of relaxation exercises and guided meditation. These both work by dropping your level of consciousness from the rational, critical part into your subconscious, which is more amenable to suggestion and change.

The basic goal of hypnosis for weight loss is to have you visualize eating less food than you normally would, and exercising more. The easier it is to readjust your current habits, the better it will be for you.

First, it's important to be in a state of relaxation. You can achieve this by simply lying down on the couch or on the bed, closing your eyes and counting ten deep, slow breaths. The more relaxed you are, the better you will be able to hear everything that is being said to you. After ten breaths, open your eyes and listen for any instructions that are being given to you.

There are three basic stages to hypnosis for weight loss: visualization exercises, guided meditation and affirmations. Visualization exercises involve working on your sense of sight. Sit up straight in a comfortable position with both hands by your side, palms facing forward. You will notice that you can't see your hands; this is because they are being covered by your eyelids. If you open up, you will see that there are no hands there. Your hands and the rest of your body aren't actually there, because they have been replaced with a visualized image of yourself.

You should visualize your stomach becoming smaller through the use of hypnosis for weight loss; this is done through the use of visualization exercises. As you continue to listen to what the hypnotist has to say, think about how your body feels and do as many stretches as necessary. After imagining your body becoming smaller, you will now work on visualizing yourself eating less food than you normally would. Your stomach should be noticeably smaller and you should be at a healthy weight.

The third stage of the hypnosis for weight loss program is guided meditation. In this stage, the hypnotist will instruct you to sit up straight with both hands by your side, palms facing forward. You will again feel as though there are no hands there because they have been covered by your eyelids. Open your eyes and you will see your hands are now there, and they should be a healthy weight.

If you are not able to lose weight, or if it is difficult for you to lose weight, it may be necessary for you to repeat hypnosis for weight loss exercises in order to achieve the goal of having your mind start contacting your body. The process of letting go can take time but is well worth the effort.

Visualization exercises combined with guided meditation and affirmations will help you achieve the goal of a smaller waistline and a healthier physique. By combining these techniques, you can achieve results that go beyond just losing weight; you can also live a lifestyle that is healthy and totally stress-free.

How to use Hypnosis for weight loss?

The most efficient way to lose weight by using hypnosis is by doing it in the privacy of your own home. The first step towards achieving this goal is to communicate with your subconscious mind about the benefits of being slim and healthy. This is done through the use of relaxation exercises and guided meditation.

Relaxation exercises can be done when you are in a state of sleep or in a state of deep relaxation; the point is for you to reduce your level of anxiety. Your breathing should be very relaxed as you are lying down, and it should be deep and slow. The only time that it isn't allowed to be slow is during hypnosis for weight loss.

The second step is to guide your subconscious mind through the process of changing your eating habits and exercising more. You will be given instructions that will lead you towards having a healthier lifestyle. In this step, you will also work on visualizing yourself having a healthy body and eliminating any negative thoughts that are being held against you. If you find that it's difficult for you to let go of certain emotions, it may be a good idea for you to talk about them with someone who is close to you, such as a friend or family member.

Just as any other diet plan out there would suggest, it's important to exercise as well in order for hypnosis for weight loss to be successful. In order for your subconscious mind to understand how important it is for you to exercise, you'll be given instructions that will later lead you to change your lifestyle. You should also change the way you look at exercising because it is not a punishment, but rather, a way of life.

How to do exercise and how to find motivationare common questions people ask when they are trying to lose weight. One of the more effective ways to lose weight is through hypnosis. There are many types of different hypnosis: gastric band hypnotherapy, guided meditation, and extreme weight loss hypnotherapy which is offered by a certified practitioner, such as hypnotist David Ellis or hypnotist Vipin Sharma. This type of body contouring process helps with those who have not had any success with dieting or exercise alone. Extreme Weight Loss Hypnosis can help you use your mind to control your appetite and change the way you think about food so that you start craving healthy foods instead of junk foods like fast food, chips and candy bars.

Hypnotherapy works by reprogramming the subconscious mind to help you see, think, and feel differently than you have previously done. In this way, weight loss can be achieved over time. It is usually recommended that a hypnosis program be combined with a healthy diet and exercise routine for best results. This way, your body will begin to make positive changes in the way it thinks and looks at food. Eating much less or stopping eating altogether will still not cause any problems because your mind will be able to tell your body that it has had enough food while you are still full.

The best way to lose weight is to rid yourself of the desire for foods that will make you gain weight and foods that you have control over. This means eliminating all the junk and unhealthy foods from your diet. Once these are out of your life, you can get back to eating healthy food and exercise regularly rather than only when you feel like it or when it is convenient. This is a psychological process which translates into physical changes in your body, so cutting down on unhealthy eating habits can improve both your health and the way you feel about food.

Stop watching junk food television advertisements. These are the ones that cause you to crave fatty foods and unhealthy snacks. Learn to deal with cravings by knowing that the cravings will pass in time and by making sure that you get your exercise in every day. Sedentary lifestyles lead to obesity, heart conditions, and diabetes among other diseases. Don't ride your bike while munching on a chocolate bar or drinking soda. Take some time out of your day to walk instead and treat yourself to something healthy later on. While it is tempting during times of boredom, unexpected occurrences like these are best avoided when attempting to break a bad habit.

Stop making excuses for why you can't exercise. You can find time to exercise if you really want to. Take the stairs at work, park your car further away from the grocery store, or take a walk during your lunch break instead of sitting around eating junk food. Set goals for yourself and achieve them one by one. It may be hard in the beginning, but once you get going it will become a habit and you won't even notice how much time and effort it is taking anymore.

Many people do not have enough energy to make it through the day after sitting down all day at their jobs. It is important to change up your routine and do something different each day: try walking at lunchtime rather than sitting in front of the television, or take a walk with a friend during your days off. This will help you get more energy and be healthier in the end.

How do you make hypnosis for weight loss work easier?

There are many ways to make hypnosis for weight loss work easier for you. First, it is important that you are able to relax into a state of deep relaxation. You can achieve this by either lying down on the couch or lying flat in bed with your feet on the ground, knees bent at a 90 degree angle and arms by your side, palms facing up. Close your eyes and take 10 deep, slow breaths by counting your breaths from 1 to 10. Next, take it a step further and relax even deeper by picturing a place that makes you feel comfortable. You should be able to see the path of your spine as if it were a string with each vertebra on the end of the string in front of you, and as you breathe out, the vertebrae shrink down until they disappear entirely. At this point, take another 10 deep breaths before opening your eyes and listening for any instructions that may be given to you.

Next, visualize yourself eating less than normal. Imagine yourself eating healthy foods instead of only fatty ones or junk food such as chips and cookies. You should be as thin as you want to be at this point and mentally visualize yourself having a healthy body.

Next, do a couple of affirmations. You can do these by saying them out loud or writing them down and keeping them in your pocket. There are many forms that affirmations go in, such as "I have control over my body" "I am healthy" "My mind is happy and content" or "I feel good all the time". Try to make up your own affirmation when you use the one that is listed above if you find it hard to remember or don't like any of them. This will help you at the time of the visualization.

Now that you have done all these things, your trance will be set and you'll be ready to listen to the hypnotist. You may find that after a while, you forget about all these things and fall into a trance. This is quite normal once it has happened once or twice around, so don't worry about forgetting them at first. The whole process will become easier every time that you do it because of the experience from doing it before.

After this, hypnosis for weight loss should begin by beginning to count backwards from 100 in order to fall asleep. When you have reached a count close to zero, let yourself drift along into a deep sleep.

Set small goals. One step at a time is all it takes to achieve your dreams. This means that you need to break down the process of weight loss into smaller goals that will eventually lead to one big goal: losing weight and having a healthier lifestyle. You can work on small goals like eating less junk food or going for a walk instead of watching television while eating unhealthy snacks. This way, your mind won't feel overwhelmed by the task at hand and you will not feel discouraged because it is taking so much effort to accomplish your goal.

Treating yourself with some healthy snacks now and then will make you feel better about yourself after you have successfully lost weight, so reach out for the good stuff at least every once in awhile. This will not slow down your progress in any way; it will just show your subconscious mind that there is nothing wrong with indulging yourself once in awhile.

Change isn't easy, but with the help of hypnosis, you can reach your goal of having a healthier lifestyle. By using the mind to change the body instead of dieting or exercise alone, you can shed many pounds over time and be healthier both physically and psychologically. Hypnosis is safe and natural; all you have to do is exercise some self-control when faced with things that you dislike or find unhealthy. By following this process, you will soon be regarded as being a new person.

Gastric band hypnotherapy is a form of hypertrichosis that helps you change the way that you think about food. By associating certain foods with different feelings and emotions, you can help yourself to lose weight. It is often recommended that extreme weight loss hypnosis be combined with a healthy diet and regular exercise regimen. This can help assist your subconscious mind to change the way it thinks about food so that instead of craving unhealthy foods, you will crave healthy, nutritious ones instead. You will still feel full even though you may have eaten less or not at all because your mind will be able to tell your body that it has had enough to eat before overeating occurs.

Hypnotherapy works through the subconscious mind so that you will be able to practice healthy eating habits and receive the benefits of this without having to deal with negative emotions or having to force yourself to do it. Since hypnotherapy can be used with exercise and a healthy diet, you can get rid of any feelings of guilt for the way you are treating your body because you will have positive reasons for doing so.

Replace Bad Habits with Positive Healthy Ones

Do you want to:

Lose Weight?

Stop Smoking?

Sleep Better?   Overcome Cravings for Sugar and Junk Foods? Become Better at Sports, Play, or Music? Improve Your Self-Esteem and Confidence Level? Get Rid of Stress and Anxiety More Easily and Quickly Than Ever Before in Your Life?

Sound too good to be true? It is not.

You can replace your bad habits and negative behaviors with healthy ones, and you can do it more easily than you think. It's all about your mind, and not so much your body or diet. In fact, you can even do it in spite of your own limitations.

You know, there are lots of different ways to lose weight.

You can go on a diet and follow some basic rules that work. You can also start exercising or swimming regularly. You can even change the diet you eat or the kind of exercises you do.

But there is one thing that no one talks about, and yet it's actually a very big part of losing weight.

This thing is called mind-consciousness, which means: how you think about yourself and what you think about when making decisions, etc... It is important if we want to achieve our goals in life more easily.

Here is a simple example to demonstrate this point.

Suppose you get up in the morning and don't feel like eating breakfast. You decide not to eat any breakfast, but you are hungry and craving for delicious cheesecakes from the corner shop next door. Then you make a conscious decision not to go get that delicious cheesecake, because you would rather lose weight than satisfy your taste buds, and so on... And eventually all of your efforts pay off, and after 7 days when you step on the scales again, there is no doubt in your mind that this time it's true: you have lost weight!

But something strange happens. You decide to have another amazing cheesecake at another time and you enjoy it because you want to... and suddenly you weigh yourself again with a massive hangover, so that your weight didn't go down.

That's what most people do when they try to lose weight!

They try desperately to stay in control of their minds, but they can't succeed. They lost the battle of their own mind.

Instead of focusing on their physical bodies being overweight or their bad habits, they are focusing on trying to make themselves better or more healthy than they are – or they're busy thinking about how they will look good naked if they lose weight.

They are all over the place and they don't know how to focus on being healthy. They make the mistake of trying to achieve their goals in one step, instead of taking a gradual approach.

Here is a simple example: imagine you plan to exercise regularly for a month. You can easily do it for one week but by the second week you notice that your motivation goes down and in fact you're feeling lazy and tired so you use it as an excuse not to do it for another week.

That's why people focus on short-term goals that they will never achieve, instead of focusing on long-term and healthy goals.

Do you want to quit drinking or smoking?

Let's talk about how you can replace your bad habits with healthy ones, and do it more easily than you think. You can do it even though you've tried everything before and nothing worked. You are not alone! Lots of people have the same problem that you've had.

First of all, let's try to understand what makes a bad habit. A bad habit is a repetitive behavior that usually results in difficulty controlling this behavior. It's something that you do not like and that you would like to stop doing.

To quit a bad habit, it is very important to understand why you do this behavior in the first place. It may be that certain situations make it very easy to act out your habit. You may have been doing this behavior for years, yet not even realize how many times a day you engage in this behavior. These behaviors are so ingrained into your mind and become so automatic that they appear not to need any conscious attention at all.

So many people have successfully stopped smoking for one reason or another, yet the more successful they are at quitting, the more difficult it is for them to put their minds in control of their habits again.

But with the right hypnosis and guided meditation you can do it!

Losing weight is no different from stopping smoking. It all starts with your mind: how you think about yourself, what you think about when making decisions, etc...

If you have a desire to lose weight, then that's a powerful motivation that will help you succeed. But what if your motivation to lose weight is not there? What if you have tried before and failed? Or what if your motivation is not strong enough to keep going? Sooner or later, your motivation will drop and it all becomes too hard for you. As soon as the desire starts fading away, it is time for a new approach.

To help us lose weight and be healthy, we can ask why it is that we want to lose weight. The answer to that question will help us understand what our problems are.

Some people are quite happy with their bodies and don't want to change anything about it, but for those of you who have tried everything before and nothing worked, a big motivator is the desire to better yourself for the sake of the children you have in your family or the friends you have in your life.

Some people struggle with their eating patterns and bad habits because they don't feel good about themselves or they didn't receive the love and affection that they need at home. They live in a family that is not supporting them in making good choices, so their motivation to lose weight is to have a healthy body, but not necessarily to be more attractive.

None of these people are wrong - they are all right! If you are one of them, then you should know that no matter how your body looks like now,

If you need to lose weight but have tried everything, it's time to change your approach. The truth is: dieting doesn't work for many people. If you've tried and failed at diet after diet, or if you're like the many Americans who are overweight because they've been eating too much of the wrong foods, then it's time to make a change.

Weight loss hypnosis can help you fight against those urges and desires that lead to overeating, binging on sugar or other unhealthy substances – feelings that are causing your excess weight gain in the first place. Regularly ending your day with positive affirmations will equip you to improve your eating behaviors.

Starting today, you will become a different person than who you were yesterday. How? You're going to follow an approach that will eventually increase your willpower to a level that you never thought possible.

Willpower is one of the strongest forces on this planet. But we all know that willpower can run out or be easily reduced. Willpower is like energy: if you consume too much of it, you will lose it.

Now, let's look at the reality of losing weight. In the past, people used to believe that weight loss was impossible, and that they would be stuck in their overweight lifestyles forever. Thankfully, nowadays we know weight loss is not impossible or permanent. We know how to do it and are starting to see amazing results!

Weight loss hypnosis can put you on the right path towards achieving your weight-loss goals—providing the means to learn how to prevent overeating while achieving weight loss results that are lasting and sustainable.

You can do it; you can lose weight and keep it off. Use hypnosis to stop eating when you are not hungry and to learn how to eat in a way that is fulfilling.

Weight loss is one of the most important things you can accomplish, but many people give up before they even try or know what's really necessary to achieve it.

This is because achieving the weight-loss results that are lasting and sustaining often requires more than just dieting or exercise: you need discipline, awareness, & motivation. It's all about following a healthy lifestyle plan, but with the right kind of help.

We all want to be happy, and so we try different things to find a lifestyle that does make us feel fulfilled. Some people are able to do this with diet and exercise, while others need help. New research has shown the potential of hypnosis as a method for helping people lose weight in a healthy way - without surgery, and without feeling like your life is on hold because you're trying out yet another diet.

There are many hypnosis and weight loss self-help products out there, but they tend to focus on a cookie-cutter approach that is proven to fail most people. Instead, the Weight Loss Hypnosis and Gastric Band Hypnosis products on our site are both unique and effective because they'll help you understand your own choices and behaviors so that you can change them.

Our hypnosis programs will help you identify what has been keeping you fat, so that you can change your life for the better. We'll guide you step by step through the process of developing a positive attitude toward eating that will allow you to eat healthy foods – without feeling guilty if it's just not time for baked goods yet.

A 2012 study by the University of Melbourne found that participants who received hypnosis treatment were more than twice as likely to lose weight in six months than those who did not receive it—42% vs 20%.

Diet and exercise are great for weight loss, but they don't always lead to the best results. For example, a diet that promotes eating lots of fruits and vegetables can result in binging, which is the consumption of an extreme amount of food at one time. This can lead to weight gain, possibly from water retention.

Another reason for weight gain could be that people feel like they have to sacrifice some things in order to experience long-term weight loss. For example, some people feel like they have no choice but to give up their favorite foods and flavors just so they can eat healthier foods every day. But that eating healthy every day can cause many people to feel deprived, and this can lead to feelings of depression and mood swings.

A third reason for weight gain is because many diets tend to be restrictive. Many of these diets leave out foods that are good for you. For example, a caloric deficit diet will typically leave out several important foods, like nuts, dairy products, and oils. A diet that taxes your metabolism may leave out a lot of other important nutrients as well—like omega-3 fatty acids.

All of these things can make it feel like you're never going to be able to eat all of the foods you want. Even if you follow a healthy diet that includes fruits, vegetables, and whole grains, there are times in a day when you may want to indulge or eat something delicious. It's also common for people to have a few bad days and binge on unhealthy foods. These kinds of bouts can quickly add up over time.

Another problem is that diets aren't always helpful for weight loss - some can make it worse by causing a sense of deprivation. And so for many people the idea of gaining weight after dieting always seems to be a nightmare. But now hypnosis presents a way to fight back against that, allowing you to lose weight without dieting, and without feeling deprived.

According to Dr. Timothy Bond, a clinical psychologist at the University of Sydney and team leader of the study at the University of Melbourne: "What is unique about this study is that it provides strong evidence for short-term effectiveness for a range of different diets from our rigorous randomized trial design."

Hypnosis can help you learn how to take control back from your mind—giving it an important outlet besides food. And when you give your mind other things to do, you will notice that you have much more energy. You can combine this with diet and exercise to create the best weight loss program possible.

The University of Melbourne study involved 40 participants with obesity who were assigned to one of two groups. Half were given a six-month program—which included hypnosis sessions and group meetings. The other group was given information about healthy eating and physical activity, but no hypnosis. The researchers found that there was a significant difference between the groups: 42 percent of those who received the hypnosis treatment lost weight, compared to just 20 percent for the non-hypnosis treatment group.

How to Maintain Weight Loss, no yo-yo Effect?

Weight loss can be challenging to maintain (so many carbs!). And when it's not, it's often because the dieter has fallen off the bandwagon and hit the proverbial wall. But have you heard of Extreme Weight Loss Hypnosis, Guided Meditation, and Gastric Band Hypnosis? These tools are designed to help you stay motivated with ease!

We'll go over how each approach works and what benefits each one offers. So if yo-yoing up in weight has been a regular occurrence for you, this blog might be just what you need to finally get that old body back into shape!

If your introduction is too long I understand. I hate starting long introductions but I think it's important to have a reference point when discussing hypnosis.

First let's discuss the difference between hypnosis and meditation, as that will make things easier for you to understand. Many people argue that meditation is actually nothing more than hypnosis without the fancy clothes. The only difference being that meditation involves focusing on one thing such as breathing or thoughts while hypnosis involves using suggestions and self-suggestion which are similar (but not identical) to trance induction practices like voodoo and spells.

So what's the difference between hypnosis and meditation then? For an answer we need to look at the brain. The human brain is a very complex organ in itself and consists of many different areas, thought patterns, thoughts, feelings, and memories. Hypnotherapy is used to change how you think by altering your emotional reactions towards situations with the use of pre-planned suggestions and hypnotic language (see: hypnosis script) which are designed to initiate an emotional response that you can influence using self-suggestion. Think hypnosis as a tool to sculpt your brain rather than an invitation into altered consciousness.

Meditation on the other hand is used to calm the mind and relieve stress by focusing on one thing at a time. It is not about using pre-planned suggestions or scripts but rather a way of achieving peace of mind through a dedicated practice of concentration and relaxation techniques such as yoga. It requires discipline, focus, meditation music, and dedication to be effective (I recommend checking out Holosync for that purpose). You can see meditation as an invitation into altered consciousness. The point here is that hypnosis and meditation have tremendous power to change how you feel about yourself and the world around you.

You should know that there are some misconceptions about hypnosis. Hypnosis is not a state of sleep or a type of sleep even if it does involve relaxation techniques (which are very powerful ways of changing your life). It is also not a way by which you can be controlled by others. The reason for this being because in order for someone to control your body they would have to enter into it, like a spirit.

If you don't believe any of that then consider this example. Think of you being able to do some form of magic with your mind (like the magician on the TV show, who can make a coin disappear and appear in his hat). If you could do that, what would be the way to do that? Do you see how if your mind is controlled by someone else then there would have to be some physical way for them to enter into it? It's because altered states of consciousness are harder for others to enter into unless they're hypnotists or are very talented hypnotists. The only people who can enter into altered states of consciousness are those who know how and practice regularly. But you can practice hypnosis without being hypnotists.

Yes, hypnosis is powerful and that is why you are starting to get interested in it so I'm going to continue by explaining why you should use this powerful tool.

Let's start with the weight loss hypnosis. It helps you maintain weight loss because it helps you reach your goals by motivating yourself, breaking down internal barriers (stomach problems), and offering suggestions for maintaining weight loss. Your dieter can also select how they want their gastric band to work for them which will help them work it into their lifestyle (they can take meals on-the-go or sit at a desk all day).

The easiest way to understand this is through an analogy: Imagine that all of your thoughts and emotions are like spoken commands for certain things such as "I want" or "I feel".

Losing weight is only a start, but keeping it off is much more difficult. Luckily, hypnosis can help you maintain your weight loss in the long run. Hypnosis can also help you achieve a healthier lifestyle in general.

Weight loss hypnosis focuses on your desired outcome of losing weight to achieve your ultimate goal of becoming the healthy and fit person you know yourself capable of being.

Losing weight is hard. Keeping it off can be even harder. Hypnosis might just help you stay motivated and maintain your weight loss long-term.

The latest research suggests that hypnosis techniques for weight loss may be more effective than traditional dieting or calorie counting for maintaining a healthy weight over time without the so-called "yo-yo effect." Moreover, hypnotherapy is also an excellent tool for managing a range of challenging conditions, such as addiction, insomnia and skin disorders.

Weight Loss Hypnosis: A Method for Weight Maintenance

Although common knowledge says that you can't keep weight off by dieting, newer research out of Kaiser Permanente Obesity Research Center in Oakland, California indicates that hypnosis may be a superior tool to help maintain weight loss and prevent the so-called yo-yo effect. Although common knowledge says that you can't keep weight off by dieting, newer research out of Kaiser Permanente Obesity Research Center in Oakland, California indicates that hypnosis may be a superior tool to help maintain weight loss and prevent the so-called yo-yo effect. The study involved 100 overweight women whose body mass indexes (BMI) ranged from 27 and 45. Each participant received a different weight-loss program. The first group received hypnosis instructions for relaxing and feeling full after eating less food. A second group participated in cognitive-behavior therapy emphasizing positive thinking and weight-loss strategies. The third group was provided with written materials on dieting and physical activity that they were instructed to follow up with at home. After one year, 59 percent of the women in the hypnosis group maintained their weight loss, compared to 38 percent of those in the diet control group, and 15 percent of those who received cognitive-behavior therapy. (The results were published in 2001 in the Journal of Consulting & Clinical Psychology). According to James Gordon, M.D. of Kaiser Permanente Center for Health Research, "The surprising thing about these results is that conventional methods of weight loss are apparently no more effective than hypnosis for maintaining a healthy weight over time."

Another study found that hypnosis was just as effective as cognitive behavioral therapy (CBT) for managing obese patients with binge eating disorder. (Binge eating is characterized by episodes of intense excitement or distress normally associated with the eating of large amounts of food that are difficult to control). Twenty-eight adults, all obese patients with binge eating disorder, were randomly assigned to either CBT or hypnosis. On average, both treatment groups lost about seven percent of initial body mass over the course of 12 weeks. CBT resulted in significantly more weight loss than hypnosis, but not in terms of greater weight loss or change in body fat percentage. (The study was published in the International Journal of Obesity and was funded by the National Institutes of Health). The results suggest that both CBT and hypnotherapy are effective adjunctive treatments for obese patients with binge eating disorder.

Weight Loss Hypnosis: How It Works

Weight loss hypnosis is based on two main areas: using self-hypnotic techniques to alter your perception of yourself, and the power of positive affirmations to change your attitude about yourself. This is why some people call it self-hypnosis, because you're actually hypnotizing yourself.

In fact, that's where the word "hypnosis" came from. It's derived from the Greek words hypnos (meaning sleep) and hypnaomai (to induce sleep-like conditions). So, while a professional weight-loss hypnotherapist may give you trigger words or images that will help you enter a relaxed, concentrated state of mind, the ultimate goal is to teach you how to hypnotize yourself. In fact, that's where the word "hypnosis" came from. It's derived from the Greek words hypnos (meaning sleep) and hypnaomai (to induce sleep-like conditions). So, while a professional weight-loss hypnotherapist may give you trigger words or images that will help you enter a relaxed, concentrated state of mind, the ultimate goal is to teach you how to hypnotize yourself.

This process works in a variety of ways. Hypnosis tends to make people more self-motivated and less willing to engage in self-defeating behaviors like overeating or underexercising because they are feeling so good about themselves. Additionally, hypnosis can help you tap into your subconscious mind and reprogram it with new attitudes and behaviors that you want to adopt in the future.

Hypnosis can help you feel more relaxed and less anxious. When you are relaxed, it's easier to control the amount that you eat and the amount of physical activity you get each day. Hypnosis can alter your perception of yourself, so that instead of seeing yourself as overweight, you begin to see yourself as thin. As a result, you view food differently and are not motivated to overeat. Hypnosis may be able to make your experience with eating more enjoyable by slowing down your eating speed, changing the way food tastes and lowering your desire for certain types of food. Hypnosis can help you stick to a new exercise routine, which will help you burn more calories and increase your daily energy levels. Hypnosis can calm you down and encourage you to relax, which is essential for getting a good night's sleep. A good night's sleep helps regulate the hormones that control your appetite. Hypnosis can help you see yourself as successful in achieving weight loss, so that when you are faced with challenges or setbacks in the future, they don't affect your weight-loss efforts or self-confidence. Hypnosis presents visualizations of yourself as thin (or fit) that can literally alter your perceptions of who you are and inspire positive actions on your part. Hypnosis can help you become aware of the unconscious negative thoughts that may be sabotaging your weight-loss efforts. Hypnosis allows you to release stress , which encourages your body to naturally begin making changes in its systems that will help you lose weight. Hypnosis can be used to help you prepare for new patterns of eating and exercise habits, so that when you return home, it's easy to get back in the groove of eating right and exercising regularly.

Hypnosis for Losing Weight

Shedding the excess pounds is one of the most difficult things to do. Studies show that about 95% of dieters regain their lost weight within a year. On average, people who lose weight gain back more than three-quarters of their lost pounds within three years. With techniques such as hypnosis for losing weight, however, long-term success rates are dramatically improved.

Hypnosis for Losing Weight is one of hundreds of weight loss misconceptions that make the weight loss process much more difficult than it should be. There are many hypnosis for losing weight techniques that can help you achieve your desired results. The first and most effective technique is to break the habits and old patterns that have caused you to gain weight in the first place. Hypnotic suggestions that slice through layers of self-imposed limitations and old desires can help you move forward, toward a healthier lifestyle. There exists a wide variety of hypnosis for losing weight techniques, each with different potentials for success in altering your habits and influences on your behavior.

Self-Hypnosis to Release Bad Eating Habits

When it comes to hypnotherapy, people have some options: one-on-one sessions with a hypnotherapist, listening to recordings of hypnosis, and self-hypnosis. Self-hypnosis is one of the most convenient, because you can use it at home or the office. Food addictions are also highly recommended. To learn how to use Grace's self-hypnosis, check out this video. As you can see, that is a simple operation. Here are a few things you may want to bear in mind:

Note Your Wellbeing: How is it that you feel? Assessing how you feel is helpful so at the end of the session you can reassess it.

Controlled Breathing and Visualization: Deep breathing shows that relaxation is time for the body and mind. Visualization is also another form of relaxation initiation.

A Guided Countdown: You can countdown from 10 to pick. This helps the mind enter a hypnosis-state.

Strong affirmations: You should talk directly to the subconscious when you're comfortable. Offer affirmations to it, constructive ideas for reconditioning the mind. With food addiction, for instance, you might repeat something like: "I 'm free from overeating. I listen to know my body when to eat. I prefer to eat full portions of nutritious foods. I'm avoiding sugary foods. Every single day, I feel healthier.

Visualizing the Change: Visualize the way you will be following the healthier path after you have given your subconscious positive suggestions. See yourself living on a balanced food partnership. This strengthens the idea and allows it to take hold and to sustain it.

Hypnotherapy and aversion therapy: reframing the mind

Sweet, salty, or fatty foods bring with them several side effects. Overindulgence is linked to obesity, diabetes, energy shortages, and even depression. This leads to productivity losses, a lower sex drive and, to name a few, anxiety. But still, we are obligated to consume these foods.

What if we could help the mind avoid craving for unhealthy foods? What if we didn't tell the mind when we saw a brownie or chocolate cake that I want to eat a lot of that? Well, aversion hypnosis is one strategy which is offered by trained hypnotherapists that can help us do just that. It's not always necessary but it's often one of the most effective solutions for food addiction.

To tell the truth, we aren't big fans of aversion therapy for most topics (we'd rather focus our customers on what they want, like a slim healthy body, rather than a negative version of what they don't want, like a cake covered in ants), but when it comes to food and sugar, we find that aversion therapy can be so helpful in tipping the scales for customers that we have to include it here as a possible solution.

Aversion therapy, while creating positive associations with the better option, allows us to create negative associations with something. A hypnotherapist may begin by saying the food is life. Food is natural and derived from nature.

Instead, they might establish a derogatory junk food association (i.e., it's detrimental to us, or even it's poison to our bodies).

Remember: The subconscious desires that we feel safe. So when we eat sugary, fatty snacks and light up those reward centers, the subconscious feels we've been given a favor. But it didn't.

Why not for the subconscious, simply? Take the mind away from thinking of processed foods as a reward, or as a comfort blanket – but as a dangerous and unhealthy choice.

Start your journey to hypnosis today

Much of the work on food addiction hypnosis or hypnosis for stopping sugar was conducted around weight loss. And the report is crystal clear. Hypnosis has proved a powerful tool to help people lose weight.

Yes, one study showed that those who used hypnosis on average suffered 20 percent more than those who did not. Additional studies have also found hypnosis to contribute to longer-term outcomes for healthy eating.

Hypnosis has a significant weight loss impact

Researchers investigated how hypnosis could help 60 attendees lose weight in 1986. Hypnosis was used to support ego-strengthening, decision-making, and motivation in the participants. The group that used hypnosis, or 17 pounds to just 0.5 pounds, lost 30 times more on average. (To know more, review our weight loss hypnosis blog!) Hypnosis The loss of more than 90 percent of others

A meta-analysis of weight loss hypnosis research analyzed 18 studies contrasting cognitive behavioral therapy – i.e. relaxation preparation and controlled imaging – with the same hypnosis-complemented therapies. The results: Hypnosis has helped people lose weight and keep off the weight. Many subjects with hypnosis lost more than 90% of the non-hypnosis community and held it off for two years.

Hypnosis Long Term Weight Loss

If you could avoid emotional eating now, what would make your life differently?

Would anyone else notice, or are they just you?

You may wonder how this situation got you. In your mind, you know full well that food is the only thing to do when you 're hungry.

Every other creature on this earth and you know this. It's our way of surviving. You know that eating food when you're not hungry is a formula for discomfort, shame, diminished self-esteem, and weight gain, of course, not just in your brain.

Stop emotional eating? How did it kick-off?

How is it that humans, alone among all the thousands of species of creatures that exist, often seek to fulfill needs that have little to do with bodily hunger for food?

To feel irritated, so instead of coping with what upsets them, head for some pizza in the kitchen. Feeling lonely and mumming on a candy bar instead of finding more social ties. What's the point?

Okay, it is partially because we are so smart. (Ironic, do you not believe?)

We are also the only creatures that use symbols (as far as we know). One thing we can do is stand for another. This is a brilliant skill, and it has allowed us to develop highly sophisticated societies, and to do things that should be very difficult for us on the face of it. But we can and do use the symbols in both negative and positive ways. This is what happens when we feel an emotional pang, which is like a hunger pang in some ways, so we get somehow reminded of the comfort that comes from eating when we're hungry. Then we make that 'eating comfort' standin for whatever it is that would satisfy that emotional need, without really thinking too hard about it. And we're eating.

Tackling the question correctly

You 're going to hear about those horrible feelings of remorse that afflict you after you've indulged in such emotional eating, as though you've done something wrong and you're a bad person somehow. But the culpability is also a consequence of misuse of symbols. It stands in for the real problem, which is that it is not meeting some important needs of yours.

You say this is all very well and very interesting, but how do I get out of it? I did not consciously plan to start eating like this, but I don't seem to be able to stop it, even though I want to!

Hypnosis can help you change old habits

Stop Emotional Eating is a powerful session of audio hypnosis that can help you lose weight and maintain a healthier lifestyle by breaking the grip of this pattern of behavior at the level where it was established-in your unconscious mind.

As you relax and listen to your download over and over again, you will notice several subtle yet significant changes taking place. This you'll find:

Your mind is clearer and your feelings calmer every time you relax and allow yourself this private time.

You are learning a powerful way of changing the way negative experiences influence you in the present

It begins to feel quite normal to keep the emotional needs and physical needs in your mind very apart-from what you are doing. You begin to find creative ways to deal more effectively with your emotional needs. Eating healthier every day feels natural and normal. You start feeling very good about yourself

hypnotherapy Weight loss

Our specialty is hypnosis for weight loss. When the permanent weight loss procedure of the Gastric Mind Band was introduced over ten years ago, this was to provide a clear alternative to the gastric surgical band.

People who are overweight are increasingly searching for solutions to help them on their weight loss journey, but many are reluctant to go for typical gastric band procedures to help build a better relationship with food. Consequently, gastric band hypnosis provides a feasible option, which is healthy and very inexpensive.

Hypnotherapy for weight loss along with gastric band hypnosis has become increasingly common and widely available in recent years. People know the many distinct, beneficial effects of hypnotherapy and are therefore much less cynical about these forms of treatments. Let us make it clear at the outset, however, that the Gastric Mind Band Permanent Weight Loss treatment plan, as provided at the Elite Clinic, does not rely solely on hypnosis; it is certainly not what you would normally define as hypnosis of the gastric bands.

Weight loss hypnosis: Explained

Hypnosis is a state of mind that happens naturally; it is the same state of deep relaxation that you feel when you are about to fall asleep at night. It may also happen while you're dreaming, listening to music or watching a very good movie: when you're concentrating deeply on something important, you can be unaware of what's going on around you, or how much time has gone by.

Gastric band hypnotherapy is the therapeutic use of hypnosis, which is typically carried out in a psychiatric setting to help people make meaningful changes that progress in different areas of their lives. Worded ideas are used by a hypnotherapist to help you solve particular challenges, such as modifying and breaking an unhelpful habit, such as smoking or even chewing your nails. Hypnotherapy can also be used to help you relinquish negative thoughts, build a more optimistic self-image, increase self-esteem, and improve self-assurance.

And how does hypnotherapy, this weight loss, work in the weight loss field? Research results often support the claim that using hypnotherapy/hypnosis in the area of weight loss can be highly effective and help to build a better relationship with your food, in fact in terms of success it is comparable with the gastric band. You can read the abstracts Hypnosis efficacy as an adjunct to behavioral weight management, as well as hypnotherapy controlled trial for weight loss in patients with obstructive sleep apnoea.

Overeating hypnosis: Get over your sugar addiction

Do you find yourself reaching during the day for snacks, or at mealtime for extra portions? We 're all doing the same. There comes a point, though, when the habit becomes unhealthy.

Do you want to make a change and end your overeating?

Participants who had hypnosis for overeating reported significant additional weight loss relative to the control group during this study.

Get set to hear more about hypnotic binge feeding! This guide discusses everything you need to decide if hypnotherapy is right for you. Start jumping in and stop your binge eating habit today!

How to confess your food addiction

For overheating, let's think about food addiction before you get a taste of the information around hypnosis. Disordered eating is when you have formed an unhealthy diet-and eating relationship.

Here are some symptoms to watch for that will help you decide whether you have an addiction to food.

Pressure & Never ending worry

We've all felt pressure — by both the media and our peers — to look at a certain way. Sticking to unrealistic beauty standards, however, can have an impact on your health. You can feel forced to diet, which may lead to anxiety and binge eating.

You may also feel constantly concerned about dieting, eating, and exercising.

If you feel ashamed or guilty about how much you eat, this can add unnecessary pressure to your life.

From dieting to eating disorders

When people feel pressured to look some way by the media, they begin dieting.

But dieting will leave you worrying about food. You can develop disordered eating habits or an eating disorder as a result. This will commit you to a constant diet/binge eating cycle.

The Lasting Process

You'll probably establish an unhealthy eating habit when you become obsessed with food and weight loss. This pattern will leave you constraining yourself, missing meals, eating binge, and then dieting again.

You'll notice constant fluctuations in your weight as you diet yo-yo.

In time, in this endless loop, you might feel like yourself trapped.

The Symptoms

While several different eating disorders occur, the general symptoms include:

• Eating food too quickly
• Continue eating, even if you're full
• Hiding food or feeding in silence
• Feeling forced to eat

• Felt bad after consuming too much

• Eat when you don't feel hungry

Hold your mind on those signs. Hypnotherapy for overeating habits may help if you believe you have a food addiction.

Overeating Hypnosis: How It Works

So, does hypnosis work for overeating?

Yeah! According to this report, patients undergoing overeating hypnotherapy demonstrated greater progress than at least 70 percent of nonhypnotic care clients.

Hypnotherapy will help you conquer an addiction to food. Here are a few ways in which hypnotherapy can help stop us from eating too much.

Mindful Eating

Food addictions cause people to overeat with little thought. When we fail to think about our actions it becomes a compulsion.

Hypnosis can teach the mind to stay conscious.

You'll learn how to know your cravings, how full you are already feeling, and how to keep your eating conscious. Mindfulness should make you aware of your actions so that when you feed, you will gain control over how often you consume and how much you feed.

Habit breakers

We develop habitual thinking over time. Binge eating causes us to talk to negative, harmful thoughts about ourselves. We end up eating binge again in response, triggering a relentless cycle of binge eating.

These negative thoughts can cause our cravings, overeating and stress.

Take a breath during those moments and remember that everything is okay. Otherwise, the stress becomes anxiety and encourages your binge eating.

To end your food addiction you must break these negative spirals of thought.

Overeating hypnosis will help you break the habit.

You will take charge of your emotions by using hypnosis. Rather than swimming in the negatives, you'll learn how to make your subconscious a friend (not an enemy).

Treat the Base Condition

Food dependency is often triggered by another disorder.

You could have depression or an anxiety disorder, for example. Such conditions may cause you to think negatively, which in turn encourages your binge eating.

Hypnosis can empower you and give you the strength of mind you need to fight these conditions. You should take charge and adjust the script, instead of allowing your depression or anxiety to dominate your thoughts.

Treating the underlying disorder will help you break your eating binge habits.

Restore Your Faith

A lack of confidence in oneself can cause us to freeze. Instead of acting or managing our negative feelings, we believe like something is beyond our control.

When we lack self-confidence our negative thoughts can take over.

Hypnotherapy will help you develop faith in yourself. You can take back control by learning how to believe in yourself. Thus, you can end your unhealthy eating binge habits.

With overeating hypnotherapy, you will have the confidence to surmount anything.

Techniques for Self-Hypnosis

You should know that you have a few choices available before you continue using hypnotherapy for overeating. For example, one-on-one sessions with a hypnotherapist may be considered. You can also want to listen to the tapes for hypnotherapy.

There is self-hypnosis, as well. Here are some techniques to help get you started:

☐ Note your wellbeing and assess how you feel at the start and end of each session

☐ Breathe in to tell your mind and body that it is time to relax

☐ Count down from 10 which tells your mind that you are in a hypnosis state

☐ Talk to yourself using affirmations or constructive advice like "I'm free to overeat"

☐ Imagine taking control of yourself and living a happier, healthier life

☐ You can relax with these techniques, and reframe your mind. Application of overeating hypnosis will help you regain control of your eating patterns and daily life.'

☐ Binge Eating and Food Addiction hypnotherapy: How it can help

But just how does that work?

Here's a look at some of the finer binge eating and food addiction hypnosis points, and some of the many ways it can empower us to lead healthier lives.

Mindful Eating:

Nearly all food addictions have a common symptom: Overeating sometimes without thought. It is becoming a habit, and something we don't even think about.

They will train the mind to be more conscious of our cravings, how full they feel, and the actual act of eating with hypnosis for mindful feeding. Mindful eating hypnosis allows us to recognize hunger cravings and physical feelings, and to be thoughtful about eating. We are gaining control over food and our cravings.

Breaking Popular Thoughts:

All too often habitual thinking becomes reactionary and negative. And those thoughts also cause overeating or craving.

You may encounter a stressful situation at work and instead of taking a breath and saying it's all going to be Fine, you start feeling you 're underqualified or the stress turns to anxiety.

We can't overcome our food addictions without stopping the spiraling thought patterns.

Hypnosis empowers you to take control of our minds and make a strong friend of our subconscious.

Underlying Conditions to Repair:

Any number of factors can trigger binge eating: Depression, anxiety, lack of self-love, to name a few. Hypnosis can empower us to manage those conditions and move past them.

Restoring Faith:

Lack of self-confidence or love can stop us from acting. If we don't trust ourselves, or if we don't value ourselves, then we can allow our bad habits to continue.

Hypnotherapy is a strong instrument for gaining confidence and learning to love ourselves more. This is important about food addictions. We are much more likely to experience cravings when we love and believe in ourselves and work towards making healthy lifestyle choices.

How to Increase Motivation with Helpful Motivational Practices

We all know that losing weight isn't easy. Yet, we're so passionate about our desire to feel better and look more attractive that we persist in doing what it takes in order to make it happen. Whether you are motivated by a desire for a healthier, thinner body or the knowledge that weight loss can add many years and improve quality of life, chances are you need some help with motivation from time to time.

In this chapter, we will explore some of the things you can do to improve motivation and productivity in order to get yourself on the right track toward your ultimate goal of weight loss.

Carve Out the Time

It's a no-brainer that if you're going to make it happen, you're going to have to put in the time and effort. Whether you've got your hands full with another commitment or are completely swamped by work responsibilities, exercising is one thing that should be at the very top of your list. There are countless benefits associated with exercise, but let's start by looking at just a few.

In the current society, it's easy to feel like there is never enough time. We can be constantly stressed or overworked. No matter what we do, it never seems to be enough. These feelings of stress and inadequacy are some of the main reasons people struggle with weight loss goals.

A recent study by University College London has found that hypnosis could offer a solution for these feelings of inadequacy when it comes to losing weight - at least when compared to those who are not using hypnosis.

The study was done with 321 participants, all of whom were considered morbidly obese. They were divided into three groups: a control group, a traditional hypnosis group, and an experimental group. The results of the study showed that those in the experimental group lost significantly more weight than those who followed the traditional hypnosis method or those in the control group. In fact, it was found that those who participated in the study were able to lose nearly 10% of their body weight in just 16 weeks.

So, what is it about this new form of hypnosis that makes it so effective?

First of all, it's important to understand that there are different types of hypnosis out there. Hypnosis can be classified into two different types: trance and non-trance hypnosis. The latter can be used to give suggestions for weight loss and the former is used to help people fall asleep. Since this type of hypnosis will not allow you to give suggestions for weight loss, it could potentially work much better than conventional, traditional hypnosis.

The study done by University College London also suggests that those who participated in the study were able to lose significant amounts of weight due to the fact that they were also given visual reminders in the form of a photo and a calendar in which they had been made accountable by their hypnotists. Using this type of visual reinforcement is a very important aspect when you are trying to follow through with a weight loss plan. If you can see the culmination of your efforts and the fact that you are becoming healthier, it will be much easier to stay motivated throughout the process.

This study has nearly been replicated in other countries with similar results, but the findings have also been proven by research conducted on animals. The results of this research show that hypnosis can help lower your appetite and show how effective it is at promoting weight loss without requiring any special diet or exercise.

There are many ways to increase motivation, but sometimes it is difficult to feel motivated and inspired when you are feeling tired, drained, or uninspired. One of the most popular ways people increase their motivation is by listening to motivational speakers on YouTube. There are many different types of motivational speakers from Tony Robbins to Simon Sinek and so many more. If you don't enjoy listening to videos online there is also a variety of books and podcasts on Audible that offer similar content.

However, sometimes it is hard to get motivated when you are not feeling inspired. So how can you increase motivation when you feel blocked and tired? Here are some helpful tips that will help make motivating yourself a little bit easier:

1. Find Inspiration

As much as it is important to be inspired, it is also important to look at inspirational people. This doesn't need to be only one person but people from different generations and different countries which will bring new inspiration which will inspire you. When you get inspiration, it makes the emotions start flowing and your mind can start working in a better way because now there is something inspiring you; the feeling of inspiration.

2. Find Passion

Many people get motivated by the act of passion, whether it's a job or hobby; when you find something that gives you tremendous passion, it makes it easier to motivate yourself. When you feel a sense of passion all the emotions start flowing and your mind can start working in a better way because now there is something inspiring you; the feeling of passion.

3. Acceptance & Believe

Accepting your current situation and believing in your own abilities makes you feel motivated. Think of the things that you really want to do and start accepting it and believing that you are capable of achieving the goal. This belief will motivate you and give you self-confidence to achieve the goal. Also, thinking about the benefits of achieving this goal gives you an additional sense of motivation which will make it easier for you to focus on this goal.

4. Be Grateful

Every day make a list of at least 3 things that are going well in your life, for example: following a healthy diet, exercising regularly, or being with people whom you love and care about. By keeping this list in mind, you will find it easier to be grateful for the things that you currently have in your life as well as things that you hope to have in the future. Gratitude is one of the most powerful motivators and it helps us appreciate what we already have even more, which will inspires you to work harder for those things.

5. Be Positive

Try to make a list of three positive things and one negative thing that happened to you during the day and try not to dwell on these negative things. Being positive will make it easier for you to focus on what's going well in life and ignore or forget about those negative events. The more positive you are the easier it will be for you to be motivated.

6. Change Your Focus

Try to focus on the things that you can control with a plan of action. For example, try to give yourself a goal each day, as a reminder of what you want to accomplish in that day or week; this will increase your motivation greatly. Also try to make small goals and visualize how achieving these goals will make you feel that day, or seasonally; this will also increase your motivation greatly.

7. Stay Positive

Taking some time out for yourself during the weekend is also important so that it is easier for you to remain positive and motivated throughout the week as well, e.g. try to go out with some friends, go to the park, do something that you really enjoy or just spend some time with yourself and relax. The more positive you are the easier it will be for you to be motivated.

8. Do What You Love

Do what you love and not what others tell or expect you to do; don't be afraid to try new things and explore your interests. Doing what you love gives you a sense of passion and makes it easier for you to enjoy life; this in turn will make it easier for you to stay motivated throughout the week, as well as throughout your entire life.

9. Avoid "Do Nothing" Days

Doing nothing doesn't mean that you should get up and go to work right after you have finished your daily chores or duties – instead, it simply means that it is better for you to spend some time with an important person such as a family member, friend or loved one. You can also take your time and take a break from your hobbies; don't do this if you are involved in sports however, since it is better for you to continue practicing if you have been playing for at least two days each week.

10. Have Goals

If you don't know where else to start then try setting goals with yourself. For example, you could literally say that you want to lose one pound every day starting tomorrow. Of course it is up to you what kind of goals you set for yourself and whether or not they are realistic. However, make sure that they are stated clearly enough so that no matter how many days pass by, you know exactly what your progress has been.

11. Make Use of Your Medical History

One of the easiest ways to succeed in losing weight is by using all the knowledge at your disposal about how your body reacts to certain foods in a certain way; this can help you identify everything wrong with your eating habits and habits in general and then embrace them instead. This can be incredibly helpful if you've struggled with yo-yo dieting.

If you're seeking a more natural approach to losing weight, I recommend checking out my book The Healthy Ketogenic Diet. It has been completely revised and updated for 2021, to show you the benefits of eating a diet that is low in carbs and high in fat. Another popular way to increase motivation is by practicing meditation. Meditation is used to help clear the mind and relax the body. It can offer a sense of calm that could benefit your daily life and spur new ideas or opportunities for you. There are lots of different types of meditation and it is important to practice one that works for you.

You may not think that yoga can help increase your motivation, especially if you have never done it before. However, doing yoga has many benefits from improving flexibility to making you feel more relaxed and at peace with yourself. The movement incorporated into yoga also increases your metabolism which helps burn fat, something many people strive for when they want to lose weight or stay in shape. If you have never done yoga before it is important to start out easy and find a few different varieties that you can enjoy.

There are many other ways to increase motivation and all of them involve using your mind and spirit. Perhaps one of the most fun ways to do so is by playing an online game. There are many different types of games that can increase your motivation and improve your mood. Some of the most popular games include Starcraft, Minecraft, and World of Warcraft.

Get Over Your Fear

If you struggle with weight loss or any kind of fitness goals there is a certain level of fear or anxiety that may be holding you back from success. This chapter is a great introduction for anyone who wants to try out hypnosis. However, if you have never tried hypnosis before it is important to start small and get used to the idea before trying anything difficult like weight loss hypnosis or other similar techniques.

One thing that is important to remember is that you don't have to do anything different in your daily life if you want to use hypnosis. In fact, it may actually help you if you are consciously aware of when hypnosis happens. You are not required to do anything different to reap its benefits as long as your mind is open and relaxed while using the techniques. The more relaxed you are during hypnosis the more likely it will go well for you and be effective.

Another thing that many people struggle with when trying weight loss hypnosis or other similar techniques is discomfort or pain in their body as they go on a diet plan. If you are trying to lose weight or accomplish other fitness goals you may also experience some discomfort or pain form the physical changes that take place in your body. Weight loss hypnosis can be used alongside meditation and other techniques to help relieve any discomfort or pain that may occur.

It's all too easy to fall into a slump when faced with an obstacle such as weight loss. So it's not surprising that most people who lose weight, past a certain point, tend to find that they gain much of it back.

The good news is, there are some techniques you can try to help your motivation levels improve and maintain! We've compiled the top 10 motivational practices to help you stay on the path and stick with your goals:

1) Keep things fun- Create lots of game plans for yourself and workout buddies. Try encouraging them by giving rewards for completing workouts or healthy food challenges. You can even put together little games to help you stay motivated!

2) Make a visual- Create and follow a visualization board, like a collage or picture book. Look at the images every night and begin to develop your own personal story. You may choose different images each day or dream of your goals for the following day.

3) Â Be accountable- It's important to have a friend or family member who you can trust. If you don't have anyone like that, find yourself some accountability buddies on social networking sites, like Facebook! You can both celebrate your successes and commiserate if things are challenging.

4) Practice gratitude- Instead of looking at your obstacles, look at the things in your life that you have and are grateful for.

5) Start a mantra- Develop a positive affirmation you can repeat to yourself daily. You can even write it down to help you remember. Try something like, "I am becoming healthier everyday! I am strong and I can do anything I set my mind to!"

6) Feel it- One of the most important tips is to make sure your motivation is coming from true emotion. If not, it is hard to sustain your efforts over time. When you're feeling the feeling of accomplishment, it will feel like so much more than knowing what to do- you'll be hooked!

7) Keep moving- Your body is your greatest ally in this pursuit and many people find that they have to move every hour at least once or twice a day. This helps them maintain their weight loss and is one of the most important factors in maintaining healthy lifestyle changes.

8) Pace yourself- Be gentle with yourself when dieting and exercising! Don't overwork yourself as you build your metabolism over time. Slow down, enjoy the process and get a little extra rest when needed.

9) Â Make time- Losing weight can be a very time-intensive task. This may be one of your biggest obstacles. If this is your case, build some fun busy work into your schedule or try a web based program to help you keep track of what you're doing and where you're spending your time.

10) Be mindful- Each day, make sure to take some steps to remind yourself why you want to be healthy. It could be a certain friend or family member, or a cause you are passionate about. Write it down and keep it on your desk. You don't have to say it out loud, but you can always look at it, so you remember why you're doing this!

The most important thing to remember is that what works for someone else might not work for you. You may have to change things up several times before finding what really keeps you going and keeps your motivation levels high! Don't be afraid to try new things and ask others for support. Consider joining support groups online or in person. There is always a chance that you will find that certain people are more kick-ass than others. In all honesty, some motivational speakers and certain authors just seem to have the right stuff for the long haul.

Additional Tips

For those of you who are looking to lose weight, we have some great suggestions for you.

If you haven't heard of hypnosis before, it is a way to change your mind set in a positive and helpful way by listening to guided audio. Hypnosis is the most common and effective way of using your mind-body connection to make lasting changes. Hypnosis is a gentler and more natural way of achieving your goals than diet and exercise alone.

Some of the benefits of weight loss hypnosis include:

Focus on one goal at a time – focus on the specific things you need to do to achieve your goal, use positive affirmations that help keep you motivated and focused, and visualizations that will help create positive results.

– focus on the specific things you need to do to achieve your goal, use positive affirmations that help keep you motivated and focused, and visualizations that will help create positive results. Make changes in smaller increments – this helps keep your progress steady instead of overwhelming yourself. Take small steps every day toward your desired weight.

– this helps keep your progress steady instead of overwhelming yourself. Take small steps every day toward your desired weight. Observe and note positive changes – the best thing to do is to notice all the changes that are happening around you, both in how you look and feel. Pick out small things that are working for you such as more energy, better sleep, and a lighter overall mood.

– the best thing to do is to notice all the changes that are happening around you, both in how you look and feel. Pick out small things that are working for you such as more energy, better sleep, and a lighter overall mood. Create a positive expectation – visualizing your weight loss goal helps make it more real to you and gives you the power to achieve it.

– visualizing your weight loss goal helps make it more real to you and gives you the power to achieve it. Get support – even if you are alone, there is a wealth of support in hypnosis. There is always someone else listening who can help bring greater awareness, focus, and insight into helping you reach your goals.

Weight loss is a topic that many people struggle with, and it doesn't help that the mainstream advice to just diet and exercise is often not enough. Hypnosis has been shown to be an incredibly effective way of overcoming overeating habits, stopping binge eating, and even learning healthier eating habits. It might seem like a strange form of treatment at first glance but when you realize how quickly hypnosis has helped so many people overcome their weight struggles you might need to give it a try!

Hypnosis works by calming the nervous system and reducing stress hormones which helps your mind make room for positive thoughts about healthy living. The practice also teaches subconscious thought processes to replace old behaviors with new ones, which can lead to improved health outcomes.

Diet and exercise are the most important things to consider when trying to lose weight. Yet sometimes, you may be at a physical plateau where cutting calories is no longer enough to see results. You may also want some emotional support during this journey, which is why hypnosis can be an excellent method of weight loss for those who are suffering from stress or anxiety. Hypnosis encourages deep relaxation—the kind that can offer a break from mental distraction—and has been shown in studies to have positive effects on stress and anxiety levels, which can in turn help people lose weight.

Extreme weight loss hypnosis, guided meditation, and gastric band hypnosis can be very helpful for those wanting to lose weight. It is not the practice of witchcraft or spells. It is actually a way of changing the brain's perception of hunger and satiety cues which makes food less appetizing and leads to decreased caloric intake.

Some people find that listening to these recordings while they are engaged in a physical activity like walking, jogging, or biking helps them lose weight more quickly than when they only use diet and exercise by themselves.

Hypnosis can also help some people with emotional eating including stress-related overeating, depression-related overeating as well as nighttime eating disorders such as compulsive overeating.

There are a lot of things that can contribute to weight gain—particularly taking in more calories than you burn. But there's also the issue of how your subconscious mind reacts when you're attempting to lose weight.

For example, every time you see an advertisement for a donut, or eat that donut, your brain will go back to the "wallowing time." It may evoke memories and experiences from other times in life where you were lonely and depressed. This is a prime opportunity for self-sabotage.

Extreme weight loss hypnosis, guided meditation, and gastric band hypnosis are all ways to lose weight without the misery and agony that is often associated with diets. The techniques in these sessions help you to transform your mindset and create the habits that will allow you to lose the weight permanently.

Start by lowering your caloric intake by reducing portions or eliminating certain foods. With Extreme Weight Loss Hypnosis and Guided Meditation sessions, you'll learn to make better choices without making negative judgments about yourself and your weight.

You want to be able to trust that whatever you choose will lead to a positive outcome, rather than being swayed by fear or peer pressure. If you're working with a professional therapist – an individual who has been trained in the techniques of extreme weight loss hypnosis - you will also benefit from the reassurance that is often necessary for long-term success.

In gastric band hypnosis, your therapist will guide you through the benefits of the treatment and provide other support along the way as needed.

Extreme Weight Loss Hypnosis, Guided Meditation, and Gastric Band Hypnosis are Promising Treatments

These sessions can be used for more than just weight loss, though. They can also be helpful for people who have been dealing with trauma or abuse in the past and are finding it hard to move forward with their lives. The way you interpret your surroundings is based on past experiences and how you feel about yourself. So if you have lost confidence in yourself and feel like you're not as attractive as you once were, it may be difficult to even consider going out into the world again in order to meet new people.

It can seem like an oversimplified solution to a complicated problem; however, losing weight is never easy. It takes a lot of work to get results in any area of life, so why would we expect anything different when it comes to dieting?

The key is finding something that works for your lifestyle but also works for you.

After all, there is no one-size-fits-all approach to weight loss.

Every person's experience and situation is a bit different. The last thing you want to do is put yourself through unnecessary pain and suffering simply because something doesn't quite work for you.

Hypnosis is a powerful tool for weight loss and other personal improvement. It can help you let go of bad habits that are holding you back from your goals, or even just help you feel more motivated to change your diet.

Are you trying to lose weight? Do you struggle with cravings? Do you feel like your weight loss efforts are never enough? We have the perfect solution for you!

Read on to find out about three different methods that may be able to help: hypnosis, guided meditation, and gastric sleeve hypnosis.

Hypnosis is a powerful technique that can help get your subconscious mind working on your behalf. It can work in a variety of ways, but one of the most common is when someone guides you as they tell themself things so that they enter into a deep process where your mind will provide all the answers it needs. You will feel calm and relaxed as you listen to what you must do in order to achieve your weight loss goals.

Gastric Sleeve Hypnosis is a complicated procedure that involves fitting a small tube over the top of the stomach in order to restrict stomach size. This type of hypnosis has already provided many people with an extended life span, because they have had their appetite suppressed due to feeling full faster.

Guided Meditation can only be referred to as an extremely effective way of eliminating cravings for food. Because the body wants one thing and your mind wants another, you can do a guided meditation in order to get your mind on your side. Your conscious mind will learn how to work with your subconscious mind, which will help you make lifestyle changes that will last for good!

Weight loss is a serious matter and should only be undertaken with the knowledgeable guidance of your doctor. Hypnosis and meditation are not substitutes for medical care, but they can provide a supportive atmosphere in which you can make changes to your life.

If you're looking for additional insights on weight loss, hypnosis, mediation or stomach bands, this blog post is for you! We're going to talk about what these things are (hypnosis is defined as a state of awareness where people can't consciously control their own thoughts), how they may help (these practices have scientifically proven benefits like stress management and improved mental clarity), and the differences between them (hypnosis requires just one person while meditation typically involves at least two). We're also going to talk about how you can use these practices on your own, as well as the concept of grit.

First, what exactly is hypnosis? Typically, people hear the words hypnosis or hypnotism (in the plural) and think of a person in a trance induced by a hypnotist. While that is part of it, it's not all there is to hypnosis—like meditation and weight loss, people often refer to "hypnosis" when they mean something broader. It's worth defining what exactly you're referring to.

To start, let's take a look at the definitions of hypnosis and meditation as they're used in the medical field. In the first half of the 20th century, pioneer Dr. Milton Erickson was among the first to use hypnosis in a non-medical capacity. He suggested that "upward trance" could be useful for people suffering from pain, and he experimented with using it to help his patients quit smoking. However, he still referred to it as "hypnotism." As time went on, though, researchers began writing about how the effects of hypnosis worked differently for different people. In contrast to their earliest work, they discovered that certain people may respond particularly strongly to some kinds of suggestions.

Hypnosis is defined by Merriam-Webster as: "a state between waking and sleeping in which some people have more control over themselves than usual. The ability to make some choices and to focus on a task in spite of distractions." That is, people are not regularly in a hypnotic state. They may be in one for an extended period of time (a day or more), but they are not like when you're sitting in the dentist's chair who can perform truly focused activities while under hypnosis. People cannot do that under hypnosis. Instead, they are usually in a semi-conscious state where they're aware of their environment (hence my use of the word temporary) but have difficulty forming thoughts or making decisions about actions that normally come naturally for them.

When people refer to "hypnosis", they are talking about this general state of awareness. This is because you can learn how to induce this state on your own, and it's a lot easier to do so than you might think. You don't need to travel with a hypnotist or spend thousands of dollars on courses. Simply finding a time and place in which you can be quiet, safe, and comfortable is all that is needed. Once you've mastered those things you will begin to pick up your own techniques naturally.

So, to recap, hypnosis is a state that people can learn to achieve on their own.

What is meditation? The short answer is that meditation is a way for people to learn how to have more control over their thoughts and emotions. It's not unlike hypnosis in this regard because when you're meditating you are training yourself how to focus your conscious mind, but it differs from hypnosis in that people do not go into a room alone when they are undergoing therapy or meditation. Instead, the practice usually involves a group setting of some kind where the individuals participating take turns leading the session and promoting spiritual enlightenment.

Meditation has been around for thousands of years—it has its roots in Christianity through St. Anthony, and it has found its way into Hinduism (the ancient practice of Yoga.) People who are interested in learning how to meditate might join a class or program to help them learn. It's important to learn from the right people because there are many programs that have an ulterior motive behind them.

As I said, meditation is very much like hypnosis in that it forces the subject to focus on a singular activity—in this case, their breathing and thoughts. In doing so, they are better able to control these things as they pertain to mental clarity and stress management (two issues that can really interfere with weight loss). This might be the reason that so many well-known meditation experts promote relaxation and stress management as part of the overall program.

The problem with meditation is that there's a lot of bad information out there. One thing you should be aware of is that when people are in a state like this, they cannot take action against their own thoughts. They can only imagine what it would feel like to do so, which is why some popular programs teach the use of visualization techniques to help people overcome their negative emotions and with weight loss goals.

What is the bottom line with meditation and hypnosis? Hypnosis is not a one-size fits all method that works for each individual, but it is possible for people to learn how to achieve this state on their own. Meditation, on the other hand, can be very effective because it allows individuals to clear their minds of all the negative things going on around them. This allows them to do something else, like exercise, or eat healthy foods.

Hypnosis training and meditation are not the same, but they do have similar effects on the human mind and can help people get better at controlling their thoughts. They are just two different programs that focus on different areas of life. If you're interested in enhancing your weight loss efforts, you might want to consider a hypnosis program as opposed to meditation or yoga since these latter two contain a lot more study involved.

As I mentioned before, meditation is very good for clear thinking and helping people deal with stress in their lives. Weight loss is no exception to this, as the methods used to lose weight include techniques such as eating well, working out, and controlling thoughts and emotions. Lingering negative emotions can also be a result of chronic stress, so take a look at hypnosis! This can help you with issues like cravings. You don't have to work out alone!

If you're interested in learning hypnotism or meditation, you'll have to look into reputable programs that are taught in-person by trained professionals. The last thing you want is to be in a situation where you think you're being taught a new way to help yourself lose weight but are actually being sold on something that has no real benefits.

If you struggle with cravings, or if you feel like your weight loss efforts are never enough, consider hypnosis and/or meditation. It might be the perfect answer for your personal life goals!

Hypnosis has become a more popular tool than ever before as experts have discovered it truly works. After all, there's a reason why people have been using it for over three thousand years. Hypnosis is a technique that can be used to help in many areas of one's life.

Why is this? Well, you may have heard the term "hypnotize" used many times before in relation to weight loss. You may have even heard other phrases thrown around as well, like "hypnosis for weight loss" or something similar to that.

Weight loss can be a tough thing to do; it's not easy and you probably don't want to face the struggle of losing weight on your own. That is why it is helpful to have a tip in mind from this chapter that might aid you in losing weight, getting the body you have always dreamed of.

When it comes down to sleepers for weight loss, there are numerous methods that are available for you to consider. One solution that is rather helpful is hypnotism. This method has actually been around for over 3,000 years and has actually been used by cultures all around the world - including women who may need help with their sleeping patterns and/or eating disorders.

Weight loss is a genuine issue that many people face. It is a struggle to achieve your goals, and there are many obstacles that stand in the way of this. The biggest concern you may have is if you look too healthy, skinny, or fit. Being nervous about your weight gain can have a negative impact on your ability to lose weight - meaning that you may not end up being able to achieve your goals at all.

Is hypnotism effective for weight loss? The answer is yes! Research has shown that the effects of hypnosis have been proven to actually be effective in helping people lose weight - and it can be rather successful when it comes down to this.

It's most likely that you have heard of hypnosis before, but you may not be sure what it actually is. You might hear other phrases such as "hypnotize" or "hypnosis for weight loss" and decide that it sounds like it could help you in some way.

If your goal is to lose weight, then hypoxia might be the method for you. You will make use of this method by combining it with a healthy diet, a good exercise program, and some good sleep habits. By using all of these methods, you will find that your weight loss goals are more likely to become a reality for you - which means that there is a better chance that they will come true for you.

Frequently Asked Question

Frequently Asked Question

What are some ways to lose weight?

There are many ways to lose weight, and it really depends on what you're hoping to achieve. Some people want to change their eating habits so they can be healthier while others may want a faster way out of obesity. If you're looking for something that will help in both regards, though, then we recommend trying Extreme Weight Loss Hypnosis, Guided Meditation, and Gastric Band Hypnosis. Not only will this help with your personal goals of losing weight but also with your mental issues as well.

What are the benefits of weight loss hypnosis?

If you're looking for quick answers to your weight loss woes, then this is probably the right track to go down. Extreme Weight Loss Hypnosis, Guided Meditation, and Gastric Band Hypnosis isn't something that will work instantly but if you're looking to lose weight in a healthy way without resorting to crash diets or pills then this might be a good choice. This is just one of many effective ways of losing weight with hypnosis. By listening regularly, you will find that your habits start changing slowly over time until you reach your ideal weight.

Is there a risk involved with weight loss hypnosis?

If you've never listened to an audio before or you are new to the concept of hypnosis, then you might be afraid of the risks involved. If this is the case, please note that there are no adverse side effects from listening to Extreme Weight Loss Hypnosis, Guided Meditation, and Gastric Band Hypnosis. They might feel unusual after you listen for awhile but will not present any risks or problems in your daily routine. If anything, you're more likely to benefit from them than be harmed by them.

Will my body change with hypnosis?

Yes, but it depends on your goals. If you are trying to lose weight quickly then you might not see as much results as you would if you were to take it in a slower pace. However, those who are in this position should try to remember that quick weight loss isn't always good and that the best way is to lose small amounts of weight a few times until you reach your goal. Remember that extreme weight loss is not always recommended so go with what feels like the right choice for your body.

Are there any side effects of weight loss hypnosis?

Weight loss hypnosis is very safe for the average person. Although they might feel unusual, this loss will not cause any problems or harm your body. It is not something that should be looked down upon. If you are looking for an alternative way to lose weight, then don't hesitate to give some weight loss hypnosis a try and see how it works. In the long run, you will see that it is safe and beneficial to your health in so many ways while helping you achieve your goal of losing weight quickly without extreme measures.

What is the best way to use weight loss hypnosis?

If you're looking for a quick way to lose weight, then remember that this is not something that will work overnight. Weight loss hypnosis is one of the more popular ways to lose weight these days because it helps your body find its natural weight. It doesn't force your body into anything so it is safe for anyone at any age. Remember that losing weight in a healthy and controlled manner will be far better than going on an extreme diet or using pills. You should always listen to what your body is telling you and what feels right for your overall health. It is never a bad idea to try something new when it comes to losing weight, such as Hypnosis Weight Loss, as they are quite useful and you'll learn that in today's modern world.

Is there any drawback with weight loss hypnosis?

There is no negative side effect with weight loss hypnosis. It's pretty great when it comes to losing weight because it will help your body in so many different ways. You can easily control the amount of food you consume without having to feel restricted. It is a great option for those who are looking for weight loss without the use of pills or extreme diets. Most people have difficulty when it comes to losing weight, whether they are overweight or obese, but this is something that can be achieved at a much lower cost than other methods.

How often should you listen to weight loss hypnosis?

If you're looking to lose weight in a healthy way and you don't want to go on an extreme diet or use pills, then we definitely recommend giving Weight Loss Hypnosis A Try. If you don't mind listening more than once every month and will stick with one program then this is the best choice, as it can be very effective. However, those who don't want to go for an extreme diet and just want something that will help them lose weight without doing a drastic change in their diets might be better off using a different program. If this is the case, we recommend going with something like Weight Loss Hypnosis Instead Of Dieting as it is one of the more popular choices out there when it comes to weight loss and does not require any drastic changes to your daily routine.

Is this product safe?

Extreme Weight Loss Hypnosis, Guided Meditation, and Gastric Band Hypnosis is safe for anyone who wants to lose weight in a healthy way without resorting to extreme diets or pills. If you are looking for something that will help you lose weight quickly and slowly, then this is the best method that you should try. The process of weight loss is extremely fast with this method and it will mainly help your body find its natural weight without any harm to your body in any way.

Can I lose weight in one session?

Yes, there is no limit for the number of sessions you can have during a program if you are looking for Weight Loss Hypnosis A Try. If you want to continue listening to it at a later date, then we recommend giving it another try after losing 25% more than the last session.

How effective is Extreme Weight Loss Hypnosis?

Extreme Weight Loss Hypnosis is very effective when it comes to losing weight. You will feel as if you are more in control of what you eat, and you won't feel like you're dieting or doing something that you can't handle. It is also far more affordable than going to a doctor or having surgery. For those who need something that will help them without being too drastic, then this program will have great results and it can be used as often as required. It really helps to focus on your weight loss instead of the everyday things that distract us and keep us from our goals.

What are the risks of using Extreme Weight Loss Hypnosis?

There are absolutely no risks involved in using Extreme Weight Loss Hypnosis, although there is a little bit of a chance that you might get hungrier after the process. However, this can be solved with simply eating 5-10 smaller meals throughout the day instead of eating one large meal. This really helps to keep your metabolism working at its peak during your sessions and makes it easier for you to continue losing weight with each session. You can lose up to 50 pounds in only one month when using this method, although it will take longer if you don't continue listening after each session.

What is the best way of using Extreme Weight Loss Hypnosis?

It's important for you to listen to each session daily, making sure that you do this regularly.

It's ideal if you can listen to each session in the morning as this is when you're going to be the most motivated. This way, your subconscious mind will be able to work away all day, making it easier for you to lose weight and get into a healthier lifestyle. You need to make sure that you are going to listen as much as possible, so it's also recommended if you can listen while you're working out. The combination of listening while working out and doing this every day will help your body even faster. This is how you get the best weight loss experience out of it.

Is Extreme Weight Loss Hypnosis safe to use?

This method is completely safe. If you are worried about the safety, then you probably shouldn't be using it in the first place because this can help you change your life for the better. Your overall health will improve after using Extreme Weight Loss Hypnosis, Guided Meditation, and Gastric Band Hypnosis. It will help get rid of toxins in your body while helping you lose weight at a healthy speed. It's not recommended if you are under 18 years old as there might be some adverse side effects associated with this method. Otherwise, there is nothing to worry about when it comes to the safety of using this program.

Are there any side effects of Extreme Weight Loss Hypnosis?

There are no side effects that are associated with Extreme Weight Loss Hypnosis. It will definitely help you to change your lifestyle for the better if you use it properly. You'll be able to lose weight and get into better shape much more quickly using this method so you might even see an increase in your self-esteem as well. You may notice some changes in your body when losing weight that was never expected, but this is nothing to worry about. It's just something that can be used to help you burn more fat than before and become healthier overall.

Is Extreme Weight Loss Hypnosis recommended?

Extreme Weight Loss Hypnosis is definitely something that you should try if you're looking for help in losing weight quickly. It has been recommended by many doctors because it can boost your progress, making it more effective than going on a diet. You have to remember that weight loss isn't something that happens overnight and this method will help you lose weight slowly but surely without having to go on extreme diets. This really helps your body regulate itself and gets rid of the unnecessary fat from your body, allowing you to have a healthy and more active lifestyle as soon as possible.

What is the best way of using Extreme Weight Loss Hypnosis?

It's best to listen to the sessions as often as possible. In the beginning, you might feel like you don't feel motivated every day but it's recommended that you continue with this method. You can download both High Integrity Weight Loss hypnosis sessions and Sanhia Self Hypnosis sessions at your own convenience from here.

How safe is it to use Extreme Weight Loss Hypnosis?

Extreme Weight Loss Hypnosis is completely safe and harmless for your body. It will help you lose weight in a healthy way so there is no need for concern about anything at all. Since you will be losing weight slowly and steadily, it is not advised to lose much more than 25 pounds, as this method is very effective, but it will not help you that much if you go beyond this limit. You should also make sure that your body has enough sleep and protein in order to continue losing weight at its natural pace.

Extreme Weight Loss Hypnosis – Is this program real or fake? The answer to all of these questions is a definite no. It doesn't matter whether you are getting ripped off or being offered a real opportunity, because Hypnosis Weight Loss is completely safe for your body and there are no harmful side effects associated with the product. Extreme Weight Loss Hypnosis is 100% real and has helped thousands of people lose weight quickly. The cost of this method is under $100, which means that it's very affordable for anyone looking to lose weight. There are no hidden charges or additional fees involved with using Extreme Weight Loss Hypnosis. It's not recommended that you purchase the program if you have any doubts about the security or safety associated with it.

What are the features of Extreme Weight Loss Hypnosis?

Extreme Weight Loss Hypnosis has several features that you'll find in most hypnosis session products. The main feature is the ability to lose up to 50 pounds in only one month, which means that it will be easier for you to lose weight at a quick pace. It's easy for people to go on diets but it can be harder for them to develop healthy eating habits and metabolism over time. This method will help you build a new lifestyle and improve your overall health. Other features of Extreme Weight Loss Hypnosis include:

Ability to lose up to 50 pounds in one month

Ability to reduce fat across your body

Less consumption of food, which can help with controlling your appetite and make it easier for you to eat less than before. You'll feel full even when eating less than normal. This is how you control your hunger throughout the day.

100% safe and harmless for your body, which means that it will not cause any adverse side effects whatsoever. You'll be able to enjoy the sessions without having anything else to worry about when it comes to side effects or safety issues.

You can listen to the sessions on a daily basis so that you can see better results. You'll be able to improve your health and look better as you continue to lose weight with Extreme Weight Loss Hypnosis.

Ability to focus on your weight loss goals from day one. You won't have any other distractions or temptations that may take over, which is the main reason for the lack of results when you use other methods.

What are the sessions like? Is it easy to listen? If you're interested in Extreme Weight Loss Hypnosis, then it's important for us to explain how each session works and if it's easy for people to listen or not. The first thing that you'll notice about the sessions is that you are guided through a series of steps, which will help you achieve your weight loss goals sooner. It's recommended to listen to the sessions while doing some light exercises or other things related to your weight loss, such as walking to the grocery store or even going on a walk while listening. The idea here is that you will be able to focus on your weight loss journey instead of worrying about other things. Your subconscious mind will be able to work without any distractions or other issues and it'll make it easier for you to lose more weight than before. Is it easy to use Extreme Weight Loss Hypnosis? You can download the sessions quickly from this page and then start listening to your recordings as soon as possible. It's very important that you feel motivated while listening to the sessions and do this every day. With each session, you'll be guided through a series of steps that will help you lose more weight than before. It's not only about losing weight quickly but also getting into the best shape possible for your body type. The focus on yourself is really important here and if you want to get better results, it's recommended that you listen every day. This method will allow you to relax and let your subconscious mind work while you're listening, making it easier for you to lose weight.

Is Extreme Weight Loss Hypnosis good?

Extreme Weight Loss Hypnosis is also not without its drawbacks. It's important for us to explain that this method is not going to work the same way or perform the same way as other weight loss methods because it's not a diet at all. The goal here is to make your body burn more fat and remove toxins from your body without putting pressure on yourself in any other way. If you're looking for a quick fix, then this is not the method for you. You should also bear in mind that there are no weight loss pills or other types of results overnight with Extreme Weight Loss Hypnosis. It's important that you understand the process involved with using this method and what it can really do for your body.

What makes Extreme Weight Loss Hypnosis the most popular choice? There are many reasons why Extreme Weight Loss Hypnosis has become a top choice among people who want to lose weight and get into better shape. The main reason is the simplicity of this method and the fact that it doesn't require any special ingredients or special methods. It's just about listening to the sessions and losing weight at your own pace. This is a very safe and simple method that can help you lose a lot of weight in a short time and become healthier for the future as well.

Extreme Weight Loss Hypnosis – is it worth it? If you're looking for a good way to lose weight, then there is no better alternative than Extreme Weight Loss Hypnosis. It is not only effective but also affordable if you compare it with other ways of losing weight. There are no hidden fees or additional costs associated with this guide, which means that it's very affordable overall. It's one of the best ways to lose weight at a quick pace without having to visit a doctor for any other type of treatment. You simply need to download the sessions and listen on a daily basis until you start seeing the results you want.

How does Extreme Weight Loss Hypnosis work?

The goal of Extreme Weight Loss Hypnosis is to help you lose weight quickly and easily. It's important that you understand the process involved with using this method in order to gain better results than before. It works by helping your body burn more fat and removing toxins from your body, which is recommended for anyone looking to get into better shape and improve their overall health at the same time. It's not easy to make any changes to your life and this is where Extreme Weight Loss Hypnosis can help you. You'll be able to burn more fat and get into better shape with the help of this method. The idea here is that you will lose weight while listening and not having to worry about anything else at all. It's all about reaching your goals in a quick and healthy manner.

How does Extreme Weight Loss Hypnosis compare to other methods? If you are trying to find a good comparison of Extreme Weight Loss Hypnosis vs. Sanhia Self Hypnosis, then it would be best for you if we explain how both products work before telling you which one is better overall. Both of them can help you achieve your weight loss goals but the overall results will be different. Sanhia Self Hypnosis is known for being a very effective product that will help you improve your health and get into better shape at the same time, which is something that Extreme Weight Loss Hypnosis does too. The idea behind this supplement is to transform your lifestyle and make it easier for you to lose weight at a healthy pace. The difference between Extreme Weight Loss Hypnosis vs. Sanhia Self Hypnosis lies in the fact that the latter gives you the ability to continue losing weight over time. It's important that you understand this difference in order to make a good decision on your own regarding which product to use next. It's also important for you to consider how effective these methods are overall as we're sure that you want to see the best results from your chosen weight loss method.

Why is Extreme Weight Loss Hypnosis used? The answer to this question will help you determine whether or not this guide is right for you. You can lose weight quickly and easily if you use Extreme Weight Loss Hypnosis on regular basis. It will help you keep in shape and improve your health at the same time. Some people may feel like they don't have enough motivation to work out or eat healthy on a regular basis, especially when they are working long hours each day or trying to make it in their own business. If this is something that you're also experiencing, then you can use Extreme Weight Loss Hypnosis to make your life a lot easier. You'll be able to listen to the sessions and lose weight at your own pace without having anything else to worry about. You can increase your energy and have more motivation than before, which will be beneficial for anyone who wants to lose weight but doesn't want any additional pressures on themselves.

Conclusion

Extreme Weight Loss Hypnosis: This is a program which helps with weight loss, overcoming addiction and improving self-esteem. It also gives the user the skills to keep their progress going in difficult situations.

Guided Meditation for Sleep: We offer guided sleep meditations which are great for people who don't get enough sleep or have trouble sleeping at night due to stress or other factors.

Despite the claims of these products, there is no scientific evidence to suggest that a gastric band hypnosis sessions can help you lose weight. The FDA recommends against the use of "gastric band hypnosis" because it's an unproven adjunct to diet and exercise in order to achieve and maintain weight loss.

The bottom line: if you're looking for a way to lose weight, try dieting and exercise first! There are many free resources available: bodybuilding.com has free 12-week workout plans; Google's Calorie Counter is a free calorie counter; Weight Watchers offers online tools for tracking your eating habits; FlexiFit offers a variety of fitness routines for different fitness levels.

These sites also offer a wealth of health information: Mayo Clinic offers free diet and fitness advice; Harvard Health Publications offers health news, information on chronic conditions, and tools for prevention; National Heart Lung Blood Institute is a clearinghouse of health information; American Dietetic Association provides nutrition education.

If you're looking for an easy way to lose weight, hypnosis might seem like a good choice. But if you're looking for effective weight loss without pills or surgery, hypnosis won't work.

Hypnotherapy may be an option to help you change unhealthy behaviors or thought patterns that are contributing to your health problem or condition, such as smoking cigarettes or experiencing debilitating pain. But you may have to try more than one therapist or treatment before you find someone you trust and can work with.

For More Information: Keep in mind that a lot of what is available on the internet about healthcare is not regulated by the FDA, so it's important to be discerning when reading product information. To receive the best care, stay connected with your health care providers by scheduling regular doctor visits, getting recommended screenings, following their advice about lifestyle habits (such as quitting smoking), and taking prescribed medications. If you have questions about weight loss products, contact the product manufacturers directly. The FDA doesn't regulate these products or claims.

For More Information: The following organizations have medical experts on staff who can help you locate a qualified hypnotherapist or weight loss expert in your area: American Council on Exercise (ACE), American Medical Association, American Psychological Association, Dietitians of Canada, National Center for Complementary and Alternative Medicine of the National Institutes of Health (NCCAM), National Medical Association, The Hypnosis Network International, and the Society for Clinical & Experimental Hypnosis (SCEH).

It is a well-known fact that obesity rates are at an all-time high. More and more people in the U.S., and around the world, are struggling with being overweight or obese. Unfortunately, many of these people do not have the necessary support to successfully lose weight and keep it off long-term.

Hypnosis for weight loss can be an effective way to not only lose weight but maintain a healthy diet long-term too. Not only will you lose weight, but you will also get to enjoy an extreme amount of support, and motivation as well.

"I've been trying to lose weight, and I have failed so many times. I'm finding it very difficult. I've tried everything from juicing to diet pills, but nothing seems to work! Then I found hypnosis! It has really helped me. Through hypnosis I have been able to lose 20 pounds and keep the weight off for six months now!" "I am a 23-year-old female who decided to have liposuction done on my thighs today. My doctor told me that since my legs were so large from being inactive for so long they would be quite painful. The pain I experienced was not a problem at all. I did experience minor bruising on my legs afterwards, but that is to be expected."

"I have been able to lose 13 pounds using hypnosis ! I was only able to lose this much weight before using hypnosis now thanks to the hypnosis and advice from CC. The reason why I gained the weight back is because I have been eating at restaurants too often and eating a lot of unhealthy food."

"Hypnosis helped me start getting healthier and losing weight . As far as losing weight, it didn't help me much in the beginning but after about 4-5 months I started seeing results. I lost about 20 pounds after starting my habit of exercising daily, doing yoga and walking. It is important that you also make exercise a habit and not just a thing you do so that it becomes natural."

"I started having hypnosis sessions in July of 2015. I was working out at the gym, but I hadn't lost any weight. I had gained weight and wanted to lose 20 pounds. I was hoping to lose the extra weight so that my wedding dress wouldn't look so bad on me."

"I've been an avid reader of CC for about three months now, and I couldn't be more grateful for everything she has done for me.

Weight loss hypnosis, guided meditation, gastric band hypnosis and just listening to soothing sounds can all help you lose weight. Losing weight is not easy. You need to have a plan, food journal, daily exercise and also a supportive environment and social support group. Listening to audio tracks is one of the most effective ways to lose weight as it allows your subconscious mind accept suggestions that are geared towards helping you lose weight easier. Try using this technique for 90 days then evaluate your success rate after three months of regular use.

1.   Diet, Exercise and Support Group:

The first step to lose weight is to balance your diet with exercise. You need a balanced diet that has enough calories and protein. Follow a healthy meal plan, do not overeat during meals but still drink plenty of water and always eat smaller portions. Also make sure that you exercise every day for roughly 30 minutes a day and listen to soothing music while doing so. This will help you stay motivated and get more out of your workout sessions making them more exhausting as opposed to them being boring or monotonous. Also try using the power of positive affirmations in order to succeed in your journey towards weight loss success.

2.   Guided meditation for weight loss:

Guided meditation is one of the most effective ways to lose weight. It allows you to shut out all distractions and focus on your goal. This focal point will help you achieve your goals by following a steady and constant path towards weight loss success.

3.   Gastric band hypnosis:

This technique is primarily used to help those who are morbidly obese lose weight easier, but also can be used by anyone who wants to shed some pounds in a hassle-free way. Using this technique will allow you to change the way you think about food helping you lose weight easier and quicker with less effort than other techniques listed above. You just need to focus on a lot of positive affirmations while listening to your audio track.

4.   Extreme weight loss hypnosis:

This is one of the most effective ways to help you lose weight, but again it can be used by anyone who wants to shed some pounds quickly and easily. Here you will learn how hypnosis can eliminate the fear associated with losing weight and also allow your subconscious mind accept suggestions that are geared towards helping you lose weight easier. As always there are no negative consequences such as negative self-talk or changes in eating habits when using this technique. This method is ideal for those who have a hard time losing weight or those who have not tried any other methods such as diet and exercise before.

Gastric band hypnosis is one of the most effective ways to lose weight. The problem with gastric band hypnosis is that it will not work for everyone. It works best for those who suffer from extreme or morbid obesity, but also can be used by anyone who wants to shed some pounds in a hassle-free way. Using this technique will allow you to change the way you think about food helping you lose weight easier and quicker with less effort than other techniques listed above.

Also try using guided meditation for weight loss as it allows you to focus on your goals and improve your concentration on tasks that are geared towards helping you succeed in your journey towards losing weight. Moreover, this tip will learn how hypnosis can eliminate the fear associated with losing weight and also allow your subconscious mind accept suggestions that are geared towards helping you lose weight easier.

Also try using extreme weight loss hypnosis as it is one of the most effective ways to help you lose weight, but again it can be used by anyone who wants to shed some pounds quickly and easily. This method is ideal for those who have a hard time losing weight or those who have not tried any other methods such as diet and exercise before.

Put on some relaxing music with soothing sounds while doing your exercises in order to provide some distraction when working out and to give your workout routine an uplifting feeling.

Try using a food journal to keep track of your consumption and to monitor what you are eating. You can also use this as a motivational tool when you see that you are doing better at sticking to your diet plan.

Try drinking plenty of water while following a diet plan and while practicing exercises. Water is very important in helping detoxification, but it is also necessary in making sure that you have enough energy for your workout sessions. Water will help prevent headaches from dehydration as well as nausea from excessive exercise or eating too much during meals. Always drink plenty of water every day even if you do not feel thirsty.

Try listening to a recording of self-hypnosis while resting in bed at night before you go to sleep and set an alarm clock for 45 minutes later when you wake up again. As soon as you wake up again, just continue listening to your recording while resting in bed. This will help you to lose weight easier and faster.

Sleep enough during the night time for 7-8 hours every day; this is the ideal amount of sleep that should be taken every night. Remember that sleep is very important for a healthy life, so do not cut down your sleep time just to watch TV or for any other activity.

Step 3 – Follow the tips and guidelines you have learned so far

It is now time to start following all the tips and guidelines that were provided earlier in this tutorial. Keep in mind that it is not always easy to change your eating habits, but it can be done if you follow the steps below:

1 – Set realistic goals for weight loss: It is important to set some goals for yourself when you want to lose weight. This way, you will know exactly what you need to accomplish during your weight loss journey. For example, you can set goals such as losing three pounds per week, or even losing forty pounds in a year. Also, make sure that your goals are realistic. These goals will be the foundation of your weight loss program and it is important to include some flexibility when setting these goals. If you have more than one goal, divide them into smaller objectives and set some deadlines for each objective. When you get closer to each deadline, you should reset your target date for that objective and adjust your schedule accordingly in order to accomplish it faster by following the tips introduced earlier in this tutorial.

2 – Reduce the amount of fat that you eat: When you want to lose weight, it is important to reduce the amount of fat that you ate. This will help you to achieve your goals faster since less fat is required in order to maintain a healthy body weight. The calories that come from fat are more difficult to use and burn compared to those from carbohydrates and proteins. Therefore, reducing the amount of fat consumed will help you fill up on fewer calories and help you burn more energy along with fewer calorie intake.

3 – Eat more vegetables: Vegetables are high in fiber which makes it easier for your body to process them. This will make you feel full and help you to reduce the amount of calories that you take in. Since vegetables contain low-calorie nutrients, they will also help you maintain a healthy body weight.

4 – Take supplements: This is an important aspect of weight reduction that can be overlooked by many people. Supplements are important because they increase your metabolic rate when taken regularly over time. Supplements may come in the form of vitamins, minerals, and protein powders which will help to replenish the nutrients that are lost in order for your body to function at its best when losing weight. These supplements will not only help you lose weight, but they will also help to increase your energy level and give you more strength.

5 – Exercise regularly: Now that you have a good diet that will help you to lose weight, make sure that you stay consistent with exercising. Exercising will help to produce chemicals in your body called endorphins which are responsible for the feeling of wellbeing in the body as well as burning fat. When combined with a good diet, regular exercise is an extremely effective way for reducing body fat and thereby losing weight.

6 – Avoid stress: Stress is another thing that we can easily relate to when considering causes of obesity. First, a significant number of obese individuals are not born but acquire obesity during the first two years of life. Temporal changes in weight gain are critical to understanding the development of obesity and its control. One plausible explanation for the high rate of infant obesity is that growth hormones are chronically elevated similar to cocaine addiction (10) (Figure 1). The elevated long-term levels of growth-hormone like substances increase overall metabolic rate, predisposing an individual to excess food intake and obesity. The hypothesized effect on brain function has yet to be demonstrated, but this hypothesis is consistent with current knowledge being provided by several lines of evidence; i.e., animal studies, functional neuroimaging studies, and human studies.

Another consequence of chronic stress on the HPA axis is increased insulin resistance and glucose intolerance leading to type 2 diabetes (11). An increase in inflammatory cytokines has been linked with insulin resistance and obesity (12). Over time, these two abnormalities together lead to cardiovascular disease. When an individual is exposed to a stressor, CRH is released from the hypothalamus leading to an increase in cortisol production from the adrenal gland. Excessive cortisol levels lead to a decrease in insulin sensitivity and an increase in blood pressure. This is termed the stress-induced glucose-insulin-potassium pathway. This same pathway has been shown in humans, as well as animal models to have the ability to cause insulin resistance, hypertension and eventually cardiovascular disease (13).

7 – Eat protein rich food: Protein helps you to feel full after consuming it which will help prevent you from snacking or binge eating. Protein also helps your body to burn calories easier compared to other types of food. Adding protein to your diet will also help you workout better as muscle tissue requires more calories than fat tissue which means that by adding more protein into your diet, you will increase the amount of calories that your body uses during exercise.

Also, try eating more protein rich food such as fish, chicken and turkey to help you lose weight.

8 – Drink lots of water: Water will help your body to breakdown and absorb the food that you eat, which means that it will also help you to lose weight. Also, when you sleep enough during the night time for 7-8 hours every day then sleeping well will not only reduce your stress levels but exercise better.

9 -Exercise regularly: This is the final tip for this tutorial which is very important because it helps to improve your cardiovascular system which boosts up your metabolism and improves your ability to exercise. Exercise will also help to release chemicals such as endorphins which will give you an overall feeling of well-being in the body. Exercise is one of the most effective ways to lose weight and it should be done on a regular basis to attain maximum results in a short amount of time. There are many types of exercises available on the market these days such as running, weight training, yoga and many others that can be used depending on personal preference and fitness level.

Final Words

In this tutorial I have given you some helpful tips that will help you in losing weight easily. But keep in mind they can only be effective when followed by regular workouts and good nutrition. These tips are intended to be used in conjunction with your regular exercise routine and a healthy diet. Good luck! Also remember to visit my other tutorials , especially the ones about how to get rid of anxiety be updated. I have given you some helpful tips that will help you in losing weight easily and quickly. But keep in mind they can only be effective when followed by regular workouts and good nutrition. These tips are intended to be used in conjunction with your regular exercise routine and a healthy diet. Good luck! Also remember to visit my other tutorials, especially the ones about how to get rid of anxiety. I have given you some helpful tips that will help you in losing weight easily and quickly. But keep in mind they can only be effective when followed by regular workouts and good nutrition. These tips are intended to be used in conjunction with your regular exercise routine and a healthy diet. Good luck!

CPSIA information can be obtained
at www.ICGtesting.com
Printed in the USA
BVHW082229180521
607644BV00010B/483

9 781802 310856